Gallbladder

The Essential Guide to Eating Well After Gallbladder

(A Complete Guide to Health and Wellness After Gallbladder Surgery With Lots of Delicious)

Brian Flores

Published By **Regina Loviusher**

Brian Flores

All Rights Reserved

Gallbladder: The Essential Guide to Eating Well After Gallbladder (A Complete Guide to Health and Wellness After Gallbladder Surgery With Lots of Delicious)

ISBN 978-0-9953324-7-8

No part of this guidebook shall be reproduced in any form without permission in writing from the publisher except in the case of brief quotations embodied in critical articles or reviews.

Legal & Disclaimer

The information contained in this book is not designed to replace or take the place of any form of medicine or professional medical advice. The information in this book has been provided for educational & entertainment purposes only.

The information contained in this book has been compiled from sources deemed reliable, and it is accurate to the best of the Author's knowledge; however, the Author cannot guarantee its accuracy and validity and cannot be held liable for any errors or omissions. Changes are periodically made to this book. You must consult your doctor or get professional medical advice before using any of the suggested remedies, techniques, or information in this book.

Upon using the information contained in this book, you agree to hold harmless the Author from and against any damages, costs, and expenses, including any legal fees potentially resulting from the application of any of the information provided by this guide. This disclaimer applies to any damages or injury caused by the use and application, whether directly or indirectly, of any advice or information presented, whether for breach of contract, tort, negligence, personal injury, criminal intent, or under any other cause of action.

You agree to accept all risks of using the information presented inside this book. You need to consult a professional medical practitioner in order to ensure you are both able and healthy enough to participate in this program.

Table Of Contents

Chapter 1: The Significance Of Cleansing . 1

Chapter 2: Preparing For A Gallbladder Cleanse 17

Chapter 3: The Gallbladder Cleansing Process 34

Chapter 4: Post-Cleanse Care And Maintenance 53

Chapter 5: Optimizing Health And Digestion 63

Chapter 6: What Is Gallbladder? 77

Chapter 7: Healthy Foods 89

Chapter 8: Risk Factors Of Gallstones 98

Chapter 9: Necessity Of Sufficient Bitterness 107

Chapter 10: The Advantages Of Gallbladder Diet 117

Chapter 11: The Advantages Of Gallbladder Diet Plan 137

Chapter 12: Understanding The Gallbladder 143

Chapter 13: The Gallbladder Diet Basics Wholesome Guidelines 146

Chapter 14: Nourishing Breakfasts 155

Chapter 15: Flavorful Dinners 163

Chapter 16: Sweet Treats With Care 172

Chapter 17: Lifestyle Tips For Gallbladder Wellness 179

Chapter 1: The Significance Of Cleansing

Over time, the gallbladder can accumulate gallstones or become congested, main to numerous health problems. This has delivered approximately the upward thrust in reputation of gallbladder cleaning techniques, which reason to decorate its characteristic and sell popular properly-being.

Gallbladder cleaning, additionally known as gallbladder flush or gallbladder detox, involves using natural treatments, along with natural preparations or specific dietary adjustments, to stimulate the removal of gallstones or cleanse the organ. While the scientific proof helping the effectiveness of these procedures is confined, many people record experiencing brilliant effects and symptom comfort after gift manner gallbladder cleaning.

One of the principle reasons for cleansing the gallbladder is the presence of gallstones. Gallstones are hardened deposits that might form within the gallbladder due to an imbalance in the substances that make up bile. These stones can variety in length and might reason pretty a few symptoms, on the side of belly ache, bloating, nausea, and indigestion. By cleaning the gallbladder, it is believed that the ones stones can be eliminated, reducing ache and enhancing digestive function.

Another large advantage of gallbladder cleaning is the capability improvement in bile go with the glide. When the gallbladder will become congested or gradual, bile manufacturing and secretion can be affected. This can result in terrible digestion, in particular of fats, and might make a contribution to the development of various digestive troubles. Cleansing the gallbladder is notion to enhance bile float, thinking of superior digestion and nutrient absorption.

Furthermore, proponents of gallbladder cleaning argue that it can promote liver health. The liver and gallbladder art work carefully collectively to manual the cleansing method in the body. By selling gallbladder fitness and feature, it's far notion that the general efficiency of liver detoxing may be greater. This can be beneficial for humans with a data of liver troubles or the ones trying to aid their liver's natural cleansing abilities.

It is important to word that gallbladder cleansing should be approached with warning and beneath the guidance of a healthcare professional. While many human beings have said remarkable results, the effectiveness of gallbladder cleaning strategies remains a subject of discussion inside the medical network. Moreover, positive people, consisting of people with a records of gallbladder sickness or different underlying health situations, may not be suitable candidates for gallbladder cleaning.

In end, the importance of cleansing the gallbladder lies in its capability to beautify gallstone-related symptoms, decorate bile go with the float, and manual ordinary digestive and liver health. While scientific evidence regarding the efficacy of gallbladder cleaning is limited, many people have stated superb results after undergoing these techniques. It is essential to are attempting to find recommendation from a healthcare expert to determine the suitability and safety of gallbladder cleaning primarily based mostly on man or woman occasions.

The Role of Cleansing in Overall Health

Maintaining proper health is a primary difficulty for masses human beings, and diverse techniques are accompanied to advantage this purpose. One such technique that has gained recognition in ultra-modern years is cleansing. Cleansing refers back to the manner of having rid of toxins and impurities from the frame, selling ordinary well-being. While a few humans might also additionally additionally associate cleaning with fad diets or excessive measures, it without a doubt consists of a broader idea of assisting the body's natural detoxing mechanisms.

The human body has its personal detoxification systems, on the complete completed via way of the liver, kidneys, colon, lungs, and pores and skin. These organs paintings tirelessly to cast off waste merchandise and pollution, ensuring the right functioning of numerous bodily methods. However, in our contemporary world, we're uncovered to increasingly environmental pollution, processed meals, and stressors that can overload those herbal cleaning pathways. This is in which cleansing practices can play a position in helping and improving the frame's cleaning methods.

Cleansing can take many paperwork, ranging from smooth way of life adjustments to based totally packages. Some commonplace strategies encompass:

Balanced Nutrition: A healthy, balanced healthy eating plan rich in culmination, vegetables, entire grains, and lean proteins offers essential nutrients for pinnacle-first-class organ characteristic. Avoiding processed ingredients, immoderate sugar, and artificial additives can lessen the load at the body's cleaning structures.

Hydration: Drinking an adequate quantity of water is important for flushing out pollutants and keeping gold popular bodily skills. Staying hydrated supports the kidneys in filtering waste merchandise and aids in digestion and circulation.

Regular Exercise: Physical pastime stimulates blood go with the go with the flow, will increase oxygenation, and promotes sweating, all of which beneficial resource in toxin elimination. Exercise moreover lets in reduce pressure stages, that could have a great impact on huge fitness.

Stress Reduction: Chronic strain can disrupt the frame's natural stability and restrict detoxing. Incorporating stress-control strategies collectively with meditation, yoga, deep respiration bodily games, or carrying out hobbies can help primary well-being.

Herbal Supplements: Some people may additionally moreover pick to consist of herbal nutritional supplements or teas into their cleansing sporting activities. Certain herbs like milk thistle, dandelion root, and burdock root are believed to have detoxifying residences and can guide liver and kidney health. However, it's miles critical to seek recommendation from a healthcare expert in advance than starting any herbal supplement routine.

Fasting or Restricted Diets: Intermittent fasting or brief-time period dietary restrictions can offer the frame with a break from non-forestall digestion and permit it to attention on restore and cleansing processes. These practices need to be completed underneath the steerage of a healthcare expert to make sure safety and effectiveness.

While cleansing practices can offer assist for the body's natural cleaning strategies, it is critical to technique them with warning and be aware about person desires and boundaries. Extreme or extended detoxification techniques may be counterproductive and may reason nutrient deficiencies or specific health issues. It's commonly endorsed to visit a healthcare professional or registered dietitian earlier than embarking on any cleansing software program, in particular for humans with underlying fitness situations or the ones taking medicines.

In stop, cleansing can play a characteristic in assisting desired fitness through manner of helping the body put off pollution and optimize its herbal cleansing structures. By adopting wholesome life-style conduct, reducing exposure to environmental pollutants, and incorporating supportive practices, people can beautify their nicely-being and sell a more healthful, greater vibrant life. Remember, balance and moderation are key with reference to cleaning, and custom designed steerage from healthcare professionals is precious in making sure stable and effective practices.

Benefits of Gallbladder Cleansing

Gallbladder cleansing is a exercising geared towards assisting the fitness and right functioning of this organ. While the effectiveness of gallbladder cleansing remains a subject of debate amongst medical specialists, proponents of this exercising claim numerous functionality advantages.

Dissolves Gallstones: Gallstones are hardened deposits which could shape inside the gallbladder, causing ache, inflammation, and obstructing bile float. Gallbladder cleansing techniques, in conjunction with the use of particular herbs, natural remedies, or extremely good sorts of diets, are believed to help dissolve gallstones or facilitate their removal. However, it is essential to notice that the efficacy of these techniques isn't universally supported with the useful resource of the use of scientific research, and clinical intervention can be crucial for immoderate instances.

Improves Digestion: When the gallbladder is congested or functioning poorly, the digestion and absorption of fats can be compromised. This also can cause signs like bloating, indigestion, and fatty stools. By supporting the fitness of the gallbladder through cleaning practices, proponents suggest that digestion can improve, allowing for better absorption of critical vitamins and reduced soreness after eating fatty elements.

Promotes Liver Health: The health of the gallbladder and liver are cautiously connected, due to the fact the liver produces bile this is saved in the gallbladder. Cleansing the gallbladder can likely promote liver fitness with the resource of lowering the load at the liver's cleansing approaches. A extra wholesome liver can also enhance common digestion, metabolism, and toxin elimination from the body.

Alleviates Discomfort: Individuals with gallbladder troubles regularly revel in pain, which include stomach ache, bloating, and nausea. Advocates of gallbladder cleaning take delivery of as real with that eliminating gallstones or improving gallbladder characteristic can alleviate the ones signs and beautify common properly-being. However, it's far important to visit a healthcare expert to because it should be diagnose the underlying purpose of soreness in advance than thinking about any cleaning technique.

Supports Overall Health: While the direct impact of gallbladder cleaning on normal health continues to be debated, some proponents argue that a wholesome gallbladder can truly effect unique components of properly-being. By making sure right digestion and bile glide, it's miles believed that gallbladder cleaning also can make a contribution to superior energy stages, more potent nutrient absorption, and a reduction in digestive troubles.

It's crucial to be conscious that the efficacy and safety of gallbladder cleansing techniques have now not been universally set up via rigorous scientific studies. Some medical specialists argue that natural techniques may not be enough for resolving gallstones or excessive gallbladder troubles, and medical intervention, which consist of surgical removal of the gallbladder (cholecystectomy), may be important in splendid instances.

If you're considering gallbladder cleaning or are experiencing signs and symptoms related to gallbladder troubles, it's miles vital to are seeking for recommendation from an authorized healthcare expert or gastroenterologist. They can provide an correct diagnosis, endorse appropriate treatments or interventions, and offer customized steering based totally on your unique fitness dreams.

In give up, gallbladder cleansing is a exercising that pastimes to useful useful resource the fitness and proper functioning of the gallbladder. While proponents claim numerous benefits, consisting of the capacity dissolution of gallstones, improved digestion, and ordinary well-being, it's vital to approach gallbladder cleansing with caution and beneath the steering of a healthcare professional.

Myths and Misconceptions about Gallbladder Cleansing

Gallbladder cleansing, also known as gallbladder detox or liver flush, has received reputation in recent years as an possibility technique to improving digestive health. However, amidst the developing hobby, severa myths and misconceptions have emerged concerning the efficacy and protection of gallbladder cleansing methods. In this phase, we goal to debunk those myths and provide accurate information to assist humans make knowledgeable alternatives about their digestive well-being.

Myth 1: Gallbladder cleaning can dissolve gallstones:

One common delusion surrounding gallbladder cleaning is that it could efficiently dissolve gallstones. While positive cleaning techniques may additionally additionally declare to gain this, there may be confined medical evidence to help such claims. Gallstones are usually formed from ldl ldl cholesterol or bilirubin and require clinical intervention, which encompass surgical procedure or treatment, for powerful elimination. Gallbladder cleaning strategies, but, in maximum times interest on selling liver and gallbladder health in region of dissolving gallstones.

Myth 2: Gallbladder cleansing can save you gallstone formation:

Another false impression is that regular gallbladder cleaning can prevent the formation of gallstones. While keeping a healthy lifestyle, which includes a balanced weight loss plan and ordinary exercising, is critical for ordinary well-being, it does now not assure the prevention of gallstone formation. Gallstones can growth due to various factors, together with genetics, weight problems, fast weight reduction, and certain scientific conditions. While gallbladder cleansing techniques can also useful resource not unusual digestive fitness, they may be not a foolproof technique for preventing gallstone formation.

Myth three: Gallbladder cleaning is a strong and hazard-unfastened device:

There is a commonplace notion that gallbladder cleaning is a stable and chance-loose technique. However, it is essential to understand that those techniques ought to have capability dangers and terrible effects. Some cleaning protocols include eating massive quantities of olive oil or other oils, that can purpose gastrointestinal pain, nausea, vomiting, and diarrhea. Additionally, tremendous people, which embody humans with underlying liver or gallbladder conditions, may be extra liable to headaches. Therefore, it's miles essential to are looking for recommendation from a healthcare professional earlier than attempting any gallbladder cleansing approach.

Myth 4: Gallbladder cleaning can remedy all digestive ailments:

Many proponents of gallbladder cleansing strategies claim that they might treatment a tremendous kind of digestive ailments, collectively with bloating, indigestion, and constipation. While those strategies may additionally provide transient remedy for some individuals, they'll be not a panacea for all digestive issues. Digestive illnesses can stem from numerous motives, collectively with nutritional alternatives, strain, meals intolerances, and underlying scientific situations. Proper evaluation and customized treatment plans are important for addressing the ones problems correctly.

Chapter 2: Preparing For A Gallbladder Cleanse

If you are thinking about a gallbladder cleanse, it's miles important to technique the procedure with proper steerage and expertise. A gallbladder cleanse, additionally known as a liver flush, dreams to sell liver and gallbladder fitness through removing pollutants and probable enhancing digestive feature. To ensure a stable and effective experience, this section offers crucial guidelines and steps to prepare for a a achievement gallbladder cleanse.

Consult a healthcare professional:

Before embarking on a gallbladder cleanse, it's far crucial to go to a healthcare expert. They can take a look at your wellknown fitness, evaluation your scientific records, and offer customized recommendation based totally completely mostly on your specific instances. This step is specially vital when you have pre-current liver or gallbladder conditions or are currently taking any medicinal pills.

Educate yourself about the cleanse:

Understanding the gallbladder cleanse procedure is pinnacle to a a achievement experience. Research numerous cleaning techniques, together with the olive oil and citrus juice protocol or natural treatments, and make yourself familiar with the stairs concerned. Be aware about ability factor effects, risks, and any contraindications for specific people.

Adjust your diet plan:

A few days earlier than starting the gallbladder cleanse, it is encouraged to follow a specific weight loss program to put together your frame. This usually includes warding off processed substances, fried elements, subtle sugars, and immoderate-fats meals. Instead, consciousness on consuming easy culmination, veggies, whole grains, lean proteins, and plenty of water. This pre-cleanse food plan allows to lessen the workload at the liver and gallbladder, permitting them to function optimally in the path of the cleanse.

Choose a appropriate time:

Selecting the proper time to conduct a gallbladder cleanse is vital. Avoid assignment the cleanse in the direction of periods of high strain or when you have other essential commitments. It's best to time desk it whilst you can relaxation and feature enough time for the method without distractions. Ensure you have had been given a clean time table for at the least 24 to forty eight hours, because of the reality the cleanse can also comprise common toilet trips.

Gather essential components:

Before beginning the cleanse, make sure you have got all of the crucial substances. These can also encompass components like natural olive oil, glowing citrus juice (which embody lemon or grapefruit), Epsom salt, and any precise herbs or dietary supplements recommended for the cleanse. Additionally, prepare a cushty vicinity wherein you can loosen up at a few level inside the method.

Follow the cleanse commands cautiously:

Each gallbladder cleanse technique also can have precise commands to comply with. It is important to paste to those instructions precisely to maximise the effectiveness of the cleanse. Pay near interest to the timing and dosage of each component and make sure you apprehend the whole manner in advance than commencing it.

Be prepared for capacity side consequences:

During and after the gallbladder cleanse, it is regular to revel in sure facet results. These can encompass expanded bowel moves, free stools, nausea, fatigue, or complications. However, if you revel in severe or prolonged aspect consequences, it is crucial to are trying to find medical hobby right now.

Preparing for a gallbladder cleanse is a essential step in making sure a stable and a fulfillment enjoy. By consulting with a healthcare expert, instructing your self about the machine, following a pre-cleanse diet plan, deciding on the right time, accumulating important substances, and thoroughly following the cleanse commands, you could maximize the functionality advantages of the cleanse. Remember, a gallbladder cleanse want to be approached with warning, and it's far constantly really beneficial to seeking out expert guidance in advance than embarking on any new health routine.

Evaluating Your Readiness for a Cleanse

Embarking on a gallbladder cleanse is a choice that requires careful consideration and evaluation of your readiness. While a cleanse can be useful for some people, it's far essential to evaluate your average fitness, apprehend the capacity dangers and benefits, and determine in case you are organized to undertake any such way. In this segment, we can explore key factors to keep in mind on the identical time as evaluating your readiness for a gallbladder cleanse.

Consult with a healthcare professional:

Before thinking about any cleanse, it's far essential to go to a healthcare expert. They can evaluate your scientific statistics, carry out vital tests, and provide steerage primarily based totally on your person health dreams. This step is particularly important if you have pre-gift liver or gallbladder conditions, are taking medications, or have any underlying fitness worries.

Understand the reason of the cleanse:

Educate yourself about the cause and goals of a gallbladder cleanse. Understand that the primary aim is to sell liver and gallbladder fitness via probably removing pollutants and improving digestion. It isn't supposed as a treatment for particular clinical situations, which incorporates gallstones or liver disorder. Ensure that your expectancies align with the intended blessings of a gallbladder cleanse.

Evaluate your present day health fame:

Assess your widespread health to determine if you are in a appropriate state of affairs to undertake a cleanse. Consider elements on the side of your power ranges, any contemporary digestive issues, the presence of gallbladder symptoms and signs and symptoms (together with pain or ache), and your functionality to manipulate pressure. If you are experiencing immoderate fitness issues or have out of manage symptoms, it can be really useful to postpone or avoid a cleanse until your fitness improves.

Review any contraindications:

Be aware of any contraindications or situations which can save you you from correctly taking detail in a gallbladder cleanse. For instance, when you have a information of gallstones, bile duct obstruction, liver sickness, or are pregnant or breastfeeding, a gallbladder cleanse might not be appropriate for you. Additionally, positive medicinal capsules or nutritional supplements need to intrude with the cleanse method, so talk these collectively together with your healthcare expert.

Assess your readiness for the willpower:

Consider the extent of willpower required for a gallbladder cleanse. Some cleanses contain specific nutritional adjustments, herbal dietary dietary supplements, or strict protocols that might require cautious adherence. Evaluate if you are organized to conform with the cleanse instructions diligently, together with any recommended dietary regulations or manner of existence changes.

Evaluate your emotional well-being:

Emotional properly-being plays a huge characteristic to your readiness for a cleanse. Stress and emotional imbalances may also have an effect on digestion and ordinary fitness. If you're experiencing immoderate degrees of stress, anxiety, or emotional instability, it can be useful to deal with the ones issues before undertaking a cleanse to ensure a extra favorable very last consequences.

Evaluating your readiness for a gallbladder cleanse is a important step in making sure a secure and powerful experience. By consulting with a healthcare professional, understanding the purpose of the cleanse, assessing your modern health fame, reviewing any contraindications, evaluating your strength of mind stage, and considering your emotional properly-being, you can make an knowledgeable desire approximately whether or not a gallbladder cleanse is suitable for you right now. Remember, the steering of a healthcare expert is useful in figuring out the extremely good direction of motion in your precise health desires.

Dietary Guidelines for Preparing the Gallbladder Cleanse

Proper guidance is important for a achievement gallbladder cleanse. One important issue of steering is following dietary hints to guide the effectiveness of the cleanse and reduce capability ache. By making aware dietary alternatives inside the days major as plenty due to the fact the cleanse, you can optimize the cleanse method and promote liver and gallbladder health. In this segment, we're capable of discover nutritional pointers to endure in thoughts at the same time as making equipped for a gallbladder cleanse.

Reduce or do away with processed factors:

In the times maximum vital as an awful lot as the gallbladder cleanse, it is useful to lessen or eliminate processed meals from your diet plan. Processed components often include bad fat, additives, and preservatives which could burden the liver and gallbladder. Focus on consuming whole, unprocessed meals to offer your body with important nutrients and resource greatest liver feature.

Limit excessive-fats food:

High-fat food, in particular those rich in saturated and trans fats, can motive the discharge of bile, that may make the gallbladder art work more difficult. Prior to the cleanse, restriction your intake of fatty substances at the side of fried food, fatty cuts of meat, entire-fat dairy products, and processed snacks. Instead, pick lean proteins, low-fats dairy alternatives, and wholesome fat from assets like nuts, seeds, avocados, and fatty fish.

Increase fiber consumption:

A healthy dietweight-reduction plan wealthy in fiber can help modify bowel movements and assist digestive fitness. Increase your consumption of fruits, vegetables, complete grains, and legumes, as they're remarkable property of dietary fiber. Fiber can aid within the elimination of waste merchandise from the body, facilitating the cleansing manner.

Stay hydrated:

Adequate hydration is essential for considerable fitness and enables right liver and gallbladder feature. Drink masses of water sooner or later of the day to live hydrated. Hydration allows hold bile go with the flow and promotes the elimination of pollutants. Limit the consumption of sugary beverages and alcohol, as they might place additional strain on the liver and gallbladder.

Incorporate liver-supporting meals:

Certain components are known to manual liver health and can be useful at the identical time as getting equipped for a gallbladder cleanse. Include components which includes leafy veggies (spinach, kale), cruciferous vegetables (broccoli, cauliflower), beets, carrots, onions, garlic, and herbs like turmeric and dandelion root. These components comprise antioxidants, vitamins, and minerals that promote liver cleansing and bile manufacturing.

Consider natural teas and dietary supplements:

Some natural teas and dietary supplements can beneficial resource liver and gallbladder health. Milk thistle, dandelion root, artichoke, and turmeric are diagnosed for their beneficial houses. Consult with a healthcare professional to decide if any unique herbal teas or nutritional supplements might be suitable for you, as person desires may also range.

Follow any specific cleanse commands:

If you're following a selected gallbladder cleanse protocol, it is crucial to comply with the instructions furnished. Some cleanses can also have greater dietary hints to have a look at throughout the cleanse duration. Adhering to these tips will help make sure the effectiveness of the cleanse and maximize its ability advantages.

Dietary hints play a crucial position in getting ready for a gallbladder cleanse. By reducing processed meals, restricting high-fats components, developing fiber consumption, staying hydrated, incorporating liver-assisting components, and following any particular cleanse commands, you could optimize your body's readiness for the cleanse. Remember, anybody's dietary goals and tolerances can also range, so it's miles critical to speak approximately with a healthcare professional or nutritionist in advance than making massive modifications on your weight loss plan.

Lifestyle Modifications to Support the Cleanse

Making high quality way of life adjustments can appreciably beneficial aid the effectiveness of your gallbladder cleanse. Lifestyle factors play a critical feature in selling normal digestive fitness, optimizing liver and gallbladder function, and enhancing the advantages of the cleanse. In this section, we're capable of find out manner of existence changes to bear in mind whilst getting ready for a gallbladder cleanse.

Manage pressure ranges:

Chronic pressure can effect digestion and not unusual health, which incorporates the functioning of the liver and gallbladder. Prioritize stress management strategies collectively with meditation, deep breathing carrying occasions, yoga, or carrying out sports activities that promote rest. Adequate sleep and attractive in sports activities activities you experience can also help reduce strain levels and assist the cleanse approach.

Incorporate normal workout:

Engaging in everyday bodily hobby can guide digestive health and promote most attractive liver and gallbladder feature. Exercise allows stimulate blood circulate, aids in the elimination of pollution, and allows simple properly-being. Choose sports you enjoy, consisting of walking, walking, biking, or yoga, and purpose for at least half-hour of slight-depth exercise most days of the week.

Maintain a healthy weight:

Maintaining a wholesome weight is important for conventional health, together with liver and gallbladder characteristic. Excess weight, specifically across the waist, can increase the chance of gallstones and intrude with bile waft. Focus on adopting a balanced, nutrient-dense weight-reduction plan and incorporating regular physical interest to gain and keep a healthful weight variety.

Limit alcohol intake:

Excessive alcohol intake will have detrimental effects at the liver and gallbladder. Alcohol can impair liver feature and disrupt bile production. To assist your gallbladder cleanse, restrict or avoid alcohol consumption at a few level in the steerage duration and within the path of the cleanse. If you select out to eat alcohol, accomplish that in moderation and keep in mind deciding on healthier options which embody pink wine in restricted quantities.

Quit smoking:

Smoking is notion to contribute to various fitness troubles, along with liver and gallbladder troubles. Smoking can growth the danger of gallstone formation and impair liver characteristic. If you smoke, keep in mind quitting in advance than beginning your gallbladder cleanse to assist the overall health of your digestive device.

Stay properly-hydrated:

Adequate hydration is important for keeping wholesome liver and gallbladder feature. Drinking sufficient water at some stage in the day permits help digestion, aids within the removal of pollutants, and promotes tremendous well-being. Aim to drink as a minimum eight glasses of water every day, or more when you have interaction in severe bodily hobby or live in a warm climate.

Chapter 3: The Gallbladder Cleansing Process

The gallbladder cleaning way, moreover referred to as a liver flush or gallbladder flush, desires to help liver and gallbladder fitness through disposing of pollution and potentially enhancing digestion. While there are various techniques and protocols available, the approach commonly entails a aggregate of natural substances, collectively with olive oil, citrus juice, and Epsom salt. In this section, we're able to define the general steps involved within the gallbladder cleansing manner for a healthful detox.

Step 1: Preparing for the Cleanse

Before starting the cleanse, it's miles crucial to comply with pre-cleanse guidelines, which may also furthermore encompass dietary modifications, hydration, and natural help. These preparations help to lessen the workload at the liver and gallbladder, permitting them to characteristic optimally sooner or later of the cleanse. Refer to the nutritional and life-style modifications stated earlier in this guide to manual your guidance phase.

Step 2: Gathering the Necessary Supplies

Ensure you have all the important elements equipped earlier than setting out the gallbladder cleanse. The normal factors consist of herbal olive oil, easy citrus juice (together with lemon or grapefruit), Epsom salt, and any particular herbs or dietary nutritional dietary supplements endorsed for the cleanse. Additionally, have a cushty area set up in which you may relax at some level inside the machine.

Step 3: The Cleanse Protocol

The precise protocol for the gallbladder cleanse may vary counting on the approach you pick out to observe. The following steps outline a elegant evaluation of the technique:

a. Day 1 - Morning: Have a mild, low-fats breakfast. Throughout the day, recognition on ingesting clean culmination, vegetables, entire grains, and lean proteins. Avoid fatty food and heavy food.

b. Day 1 - Evening: Consume a mild dinner early inside the middle of the night. Afterward, chorus from consuming or ingesting some thing for at least hours earlier than the cleanse.

c. Day 1 - Night: Mix the Epsom salt with water as regular with the instructions supplied. Typically, you may consume a specific quantity of Epsom salt answer at two separate periods in the path of the midnight. This permits loosen up the bile ducts and allows the release of bile.

d. Day 2 - Morning: Drink the second one dose of the Epsom salt solution in keeping with the supplied instructions.

e. Day 2 - Morning to Afternoon: Wait for a few hours earlier than consuming a few aspect. During this time, you can enjoy bowel movements, which might be a ordinary part of the cleanse manner.

f. Day 2 - Evening: Mix the olive oil with sparkling citrus juice. Consume the mixture progressively over a particular duration, generally internal a 30-minute window. This aggregate is concept to help stimulate the gallbladder and promote the discharge of bile.

g. Day 2 - Bedtime: After ingesting the olive oil and citrus combination, lie down on your proper side along with your knees drawn within the route of your chest. Remain on this feature for at the least half of-hour or as advocated with the aid of manner of the proper protocol you're following.

Step four: Post-Cleanse Care

After finishing the gallbladder cleanse, it's miles vital to provide your frame time to rest and get better. Allow yourself an afternoon or of moderate sports activities, as you can experience fatigued or enjoy bowel moves as a part of the cleansing manner. Maintain a healthful eating regimen and keep to help liver fitness with nutritious materials and manner of existence conduct.

The gallbladder cleaning manner can be a useful way to assist liver and gallbladder health. By following the critical preparations, accumulating the required additives, and adhering to the specific cleanse protocol, you could adopt a healthy detox. However, it's far important to talk over with a healthcare professional in advance than beginning any new fitness routine and to ensure the gallbladder cleanse is suitable on your character desires.

Understanding the Cleansing Protocol

Understanding the cleaning protocol is vital earlier than embarking on a gallbladder cleanse. The protocol outlines the precise steps and commands to conform with inside the direction of the cleanse, ensuring a secure and effective cleaning method. By familiarizing your self with the cleansing protocol, you can technique the cleanse with self perception and maximize its functionality blessings. In this section, we are able to delve into the crucial factor elements of a everyday gallbladder cleansing protocol.

Pre-Cleanse Preparations:

Before starting off the cleanse, it's miles vital to prepare your frame very well. This normally consists of following particular dietary pointers, hydrating well, and every now and then incorporating herbal nutritional nutritional supplements. Preparing your body permits optimize liver and gallbladder feature, considering a extra effective cleanse. Consult with a healthcare expert or follow a good cleanse program for unique pre-cleanse commands.

Selection of Cleansing Method:

There are numerous gallbladder cleansing strategies to be had, and it's miles vital to pick out one that aligns collectively collectively together with your alternatives and health goals. Common techniques contain the use of a mixture of natural materials like olive oil, citrus juice, and Epsom salt. Each technique might also moreover have considered considered one of a type variations in the portions and timing of the substances, so carefully look at and apprehend the instructions in advance than proceeding.

Timing of the Cleanse:

Timing plays a vital characteristic within the fulfillment of the gallbladder cleanse. Most protocols recommend selecting a time while you could devote a complete day to the machine with out interruptions or responsibilities. It is regularly maximum top notch to provoke the cleanse on a weekend or at the same time as you may have a day off art work, contemplating rest and rest for the duration of and after the cleanse.

Epsom Salt Solution:

The cleaning protocol typically consists of the use of an Epsom salt answer. Epsom salt lets in loosen up the bile ducts and facilitates the release of bile from the gallbladder. It is normally fed on in particular portions at prescribed periods, normally inside the night time earlier than the principle a part of the cleanse. Carefully follow the commands for blending and ingesting the Epsom salt solution.

Olive Oil and Citrus Juice Mixture:

The centerpiece of the gallbladder cleanse is a combination of olive oil and citrus juice. This combination is assumed to stimulate the gallbladder contractions and encourage the discharge of gathered bile and pollution. The mixture is normally ate up inside the night, following a particular timeline furnished inside the protocol. It is essential to select out superb, natural olive oil and freshly squeezed citrus juice for the excellent results.

Rest and Positioning:

After consuming the olive oil and citrus juice aggregate, it's miles crucial to relaxation and expect a specific characteristic to beneficial resource the cleanse way. Most protocols recommend mendacity down for your right component collectively along with your knees drawn in the direction of your chest for a designated duration, commonly 1/2-hour or as one of a kind inside the instructions. This role permits facilitate the drift of bile and its eventual elimination.

Post-Cleanse Care:

Once the cleanse is complete, it is essential to ease returned into ordinary ingesting step by step. Start with mild, with out problems digestible components and regularly reintroduce regular food. Focus on a healthy, balanced weight loss program and preserve desirable hydration to help ongoing liver and gallbladder health. Allow your frame time to rest and get higher after the cleanse, and communicate with a healthcare professional for post-cleanse guidance.

Understanding the cleansing protocol is crucial for a a success gallbladder cleanse. By familiarizing your self with the pre-cleanse arrangements, choosing a suitable cleansing technique, following the prescribed timing, incorporating the Epsom salt solution, ingesting the olive oil and citrus juice aggregate, adopting the endorsed resting feature, and walking in the course of placed up-cleanse care, you can optimize the effectiveness of the cleanse and aid your liver and gallbladder fitness. Remember to are searching for recommendation from a healthcare professional earlier than beginning any new health ordinary and to make certain the cleansing protocol aligns in conjunction with your individual desires.

Selecting the Right Cleansing Method for You

Choosing the proper cleansing technique is a crucial step in embarking on a gallbladder cleanse. With severa strategies to be had, it's critical to pick one that fits your options, fitness needs, and comfort level. Each method may moreover have certainly one of a type substances, instructions, and predicted outcomes. In this segment, we can discover factors to undergo in thoughts while choosing the right gallbladder cleaning approach for you.

Research and Understand Different Methods:

Start through using coming across and familiarizing yourself with the only of a type gallbladder cleaning strategies to be had. Explore expert assets, books, online boards, and speak over with healthcare professionals or skilled people who've handed via gallbladder cleanses. Gain an understanding of the components, instructions, and capacity blessings or risks associated with each method.

Consider Personal Health Factors:

Take under attention your individual health factors even as deciding on a cleansing method. If you have got were given any pre-modern fitness situations, allergic reactions, or sensitivities, it's essential to choose a way that aligns together together with your precise dreams. Certain cleaning techniques can be more appropriate for human beings with sure health conditions, whilst others also can pose risks or headaches. Consult with a healthcare expert in advance than beginning any cleansing protocol, specially if you have underlying health troubles.

Assess Comfort Level and Preferences:

Consider your consolation degree and private options at the same time as choosing a cleansing approach. Some techniques can also include consuming specific additives or combinations that you discover more palatable or tolerable. Others can also require unique dietary changes or rules that align together together together with your way of existence. Select a method that you are feeling cushty with and confident in executing, as this may contribute to a extra a achievement cleanse enjoy.

Review Testimonials and Experiences:

Reading testimonials and private reports of human beings who've long gone thru splendid gallbladder cleaning strategies can provide treasured insights. Take have a take a look at of common memories, potential advantages, and any problems or annoying conditions said through others. However, recall that character opinions can also vary, and it's important to method testimonials with an open thoughts and gather pretty some views in advance than you make a decision.

Seek Professional Guidance:

If you are unsure approximately which cleaning approach to pick or have unique health problems, it's miles mainly encouraged to are searching for professional steerage. Consult with a certified healthcare professional, together with a naturopathic clinical physician or purposeful remedy practitioner, who can offer customized recommendation primarily based to your health statistics and person dreams. They will permit you to navigate the available options and decide the great technique for you.

Consider Long-Term Lifestyle Changes:

While gallbladder cleansing can provide short-time period blessings, it's far crucial to undergo in thoughts prolonged-term manner of existence modifications to manual commonplace liver and gallbladder health. Evaluate whether or now not the chosen cleansing approach aligns with sustainable manner of existence modifications you may include beyond the cleanse. Focus on adopting a balanced, entire food-based totally definitely actually weight loss program, everyday bodily hobby, stress manage, and healthful conduct that sell most beneficial liver and gallbladder feature.

Selecting the proper cleaning technique in your gallbladder cleanse is a important preference that want to be based totally on thorough studies, private fitness elements, comfort degree, options, testimonials, and professional guidance. By thinking about the ones factors, you could choose out out a way that aligns collectively together with your desires and embark on a cleansing journey that allows your liver and gallbladder health.

Remember, a gallbladder cleanse want to constantly be completed under professional steerage, in particular if you have underlying fitness conditions or troubles.

Step-thru-Step Guide to a Successful Gallbladder Cleanse

Embarking on a gallbladder cleanse may be an effective manner to beneficial resource liver and gallbladder health, decorate digestion, and promote everyday nicely-being. A successful cleanse calls for cautious planning, training, and adherence to a step-with the aid of-step tool. In this section, we are capable of offer a complete manual outlining the critical steps for a a achievement gallbladder cleanse.

Step 1: Consult with a Healthcare Professional:

Before starting a gallbladder cleanse, it is vital to talk about with a healthcare expert, particularly when you have any underlying health conditions or are taking medicinal drugs. They can provide steerage, test your suitability for a cleanse, and cope with any issues or questions you may have.

Step 2: Pre-Cleanse Preparation:

Prepare your frame for the cleanse with the aid of following particular pre-cleanse pointers. This normally includes making dietary modifications, which encompass reducing the consumption of processed elements, delicate sugars, and terrible fats. Increase your consumption of easy culmination, veggies, complete grains, and lean proteins. Hydrate very well via the use of consuming plenty of water in some unspecified time in the future of the day. Consider incorporating liver-supporting herbs or dietary supplements as encouraged thru your healthcare professional.

Step three: Choose a Cleansing Method:

Select a gallbladder cleaning technique that aligns together along side your choices, health desires, and comfort level. There are severa strategies available, which includes those concerning olive oil, citrus juice, and Epsom salt. Research and understand the appropriate commands, elements, and functionality benefits or dangers related to each method. Consider in search of expert advice to determine the most appropriate approach for you.

Step 4: Gather the Necessary Supplies:

Once you have got got decided on a cleansing approach, acquire all the vital resources. This may also encompass natural olive oil, glowing citrus juice (together with lemon or grapefruit), Epsom salt, and any extra additives or nutritional dietary supplements required for your preferred approach. Ensure you have the substances organized earlier than beginning the cleanse.

Step five: Select the Right Timing:

Choose a time for the cleanse at the same time as you can devote a entire day to the method with out interruptions or responsibilities. It is frequently advocated to start the cleanse on a weekend or when you have a break day artwork to permit for rest and rest in a few unspecified time inside the destiny of and after the cleanse.

Step 6: Follow the Cleanse Protocol:

Follow the specific commands outlined in your chosen cleaning technique. This typically consists of eating a specific series of materials, inclusive of the Epsom salt solution, olive oil, and citrus juice combination, at distinct instances. Pay near hobby to the encouraged quantities, timings, and any more commands provided. Maintain a peaceful and cushty surroundings at a few level in the cleanse.

Step 7: Rest and Allow for Elimination:

After ingesting the olive oil and citrus juice mixture, lie right down to your proper aspect at the side of your knees drawn closer to your chest. This role enables facilitate the go together with the glide of bile and enables its removal. Remain on this function for at the least half-hour or as recommended via your preferred cleaning method.

Step 8: Post-Cleanse Care:

After finishing the cleanse, gradually reintroduce everyday meals into your diet plan. Start with light, consequences digestible food and frequently transition all over again to a balanced, nutrient-dense weight-reduction plan. Stay properly-hydrated and preserve to prioritize healthful manner of life behavior, together with ordinary workout, pressure control, and good enough sleep.

Chapter 4: Post-Cleanse Care And Maintenance

Completing a gallbladder cleanse is an critical step in helping your liver and gallbladder health. However, it's far in addition crucial to cognizance on put up-cleanse care and safety to optimize the benefits and preserve a healthful gallbladder feature. In this phase, we are able to discover vital hints and strategies for submit-cleanse care and extended-time period safety of your gallbladder fitness.

Gradual Transition to Regular Diet:

After the cleanse, it is critical to reintroduce food often into your food plan. Start with moderate, with out issues digestible meals at the side of steamed veggies, soups, and lean proteins. Avoid heavy, fried, or processed meals that can strain the digestive machine. Slowly reintroduce food while being attentive to any sensitivities or reactions your body can also moreover have. Aim for a balanced diet which encompass complete substances, masses of fruits and vegetables, healthful fat, and lean proteins.

Hydration and Healthy Fluid Intake:

Maintain nicely hydration to manual your gallbladder and not unusual digestive health. Drink an top enough quantity of water in the course of the day, aiming for at the least 8 glasses (sixty 4 oz.) or extra, relying on your person wishes. Staying hydrated helps prevent the formation of gallstones and promotes the smooth go along with the float of bile.

Dietary Considerations:

Incorporate food that sell gallbladder fitness into your every day diet regime. Include fiber-rich components along side end result, vegetables, entire grains, and legumes to assist everyday bowel movements and save you constipation. Opt for wholesome fat, which includes avocados, nuts, seeds, and olive oil, that can promote the manufacturing and drift of healthful bile. Limit or avoid meals which may be excessive in saturated fat, processed sugars, and artificial components, as they're able to burden the liver and gallbladder.

Regular Physical Activity:

Engage in ordinary physical hobby to guide typical digestive health and maintain a healthful weight. Exercise lets in stimulate digestion, promotes the movement of blood and lymph fluids, and aids within the elimination of pollution. Aim for at the least half-hour of mild-intensity exercising, which includes brisk on foot, strolling, cycling, or yoga, maximum days of the week. Consult with a healthcare professional in advance than starting any new workout regimen, mainly if you have any underlying health situations.

Stress Management:

Chronic pressure need to have a terrible impact on gallbladder feature and regular digestive fitness. Practice stress management techniques collectively with deep respiration carrying events, meditation, yoga, or accomplishing pastimes and sports activities that assist you lighten up and unwind. Prioritize self-care and discover time for sports that supply you pleasure and reduce strain levels.

Maintain a Healthy Weight:

Maintaining a healthy weight is important for maximum suitable gallbladder feature. Excess weight, particularly during the middle, can increase the danger of gallstone formation and disrupt bile glide. Focus on adopting a balanced healthy dietweight-reduction plan and tasty in everyday bodily activity to achieve and preserve a wholesome weight.

Regular Check-ups:

Schedule ordinary test-u.S.A.With your healthcare expert to display your gallbladder fitness and famous properly-being. They can perform normal exams and critiques to assess your liver and gallbladder feature and offer steerage on any vital changes or extra help.

Consider Liver and Gallbladder Supporting Supplements:

Discuss together along side your healthcare professional approximately incorporating liver and gallbladder supporting nutritional dietary supplements into your positioned up-cleanse ordinary. These can also embody natural treatments collectively with milk thistle, dandelion root, turmeric, or artichoke extract, that could help liver cleansing and bile manufacturing. However, always communicate over with a healthcare professional earlier than which encompass any dietary nutritional supplements for your normal to make certain they'll be secure and suitable for your man or woman dreams.

Post-cleanse care and protection are essential for preserving the blessings of a gallbladder cleanse and selling prolonged-time period gallbladder fitness. By incorporating those strategies, including slow dietary transitions, wholesome hydration, everyday bodily hobby, pressure manage, and regular take a look at-ups, you may aid your gallbladder's feature and preferred well-being. Remember to go to a healthcare expert for personalized steerage and recommendation based on your precise health wishes.

Recovering from the Gallbladder Cleanse

Completing a gallbladder cleanse is an crucial step in selling liver and gallbladder fitness. After the cleanse, it's miles essential to prioritize publish-cleanse recuperation to permit your frame to recalibrate and regain balance. In this section, we will explore important pointers for a smooth healing from a gallbladder cleanse, making sure your body receives the care and manual it goals all through this section.

Hydration and Gentle Nutrition:

During the recuperation section, prioritize hydration to flush out pollution and guide the frame's natural detoxification strategies.

Drink adequate quantities of water in a few unspecified time inside the destiny of the day and include hydrating fluids like herbal teas or infused water. Gradually reintroduce nourishing, clean-to-digest food on the facet of soups, broths, steamed vegetables, and lean proteins. Avoid heavy, processed, or greasy additives which could pressure your digestive tool and choose nutrient-dense, complete food.

Rest and Relaxation:

Rest is crucial for allowing your frame to recover and regenerate. Ensure you get masses of sleep and create a calming environment to aid deep relaxation. Incorporate relaxation techniques like meditation, deep respiratory sporting occasions, or moderate yoga to reduce pressure and promote standard properly-being. Listen on your frame's alerts and take breaks at the same time as had to recharge and rejuvenate.

Support Digestion:

After a gallbladder cleanse, your digestive machine can also require more guide. Consider incorporating digestive aids which encompass digestive enzymes or probiotics to enhance digestion and nutrient absorption. These supplements can help your frame in breaking down meals and selling a healthy gut surroundings. Consult with a healthcare professional for custom designed hints primarily based on your specific desires.

Gradual Reintroduction of Foods:

As you get over the cleanse, reintroduce meals step by step to allow your frame to alter and prevent any digestive pain. Start with small quantities of without difficulty digestible materials and take a look at how your frame responds. If you enjoy any terrible reactions or sensitivities, understand the triggering food and avoid them until your digestive tool has virtually recovered.

Gentle Physical Activity:

Engaging in mild physical hobby can assist your recovery via the usage of enhancing blood go with the flow, selling lymphatic glide, and boosting your ordinary strength stages. Incorporate low-impact sports sports which consist of strolling, slight stretching, or yoga. Avoid immoderate workout routines or strenuous sports activities activities proper away after the cleanse, as your body also can however be in a kingdom of recalibration.

Maintain Healthy Habits:

To hold the benefits of the gallbladder cleanse, preserve healthful behavior that help liver and gallbladder health. Continue to prioritize a balanced diet wealthy in fruits, greens, complete grains, and lean proteins. Stay hydrated, manage pressure correctly, and interact in normal physical hobby. These behavior make contributions to ongoing properly-being and assist save you the formation of gallstones inside the destiny.

Monitor Your Body's Response:

Pay interest to how your frame responds at some diploma in the recuperation section. Notice any upgrades in digestion, strength levels, or ordinary well-being. Keep a journal to music your development, noting any observations or changes. If you enjoy continual or concerning signs and symptoms and symptoms, communicate with a healthcare expert for further assessment.

Recovering from a gallbladder cleanse calls for moderate care, attention, and guide for your frame's restoration way. By specializing in hydration, gentle nutrients, rest, and relaxation, helping digestion, slow food reintroduction, mild physical activity, and maintaining healthy conduct, you could facilitate a easy recuperation and preserve the benefits of the cleanse. Listen on your frame's dreams and communicate over with a healthcare expert for customized guidance along your recovery adventure.

Chapter 5: Optimizing Health And Digestion

The gallbladder plays a critical feature in digestion by the usage of storing and releasing bile, a substance that aids inside the breakdown and absorption of nutritional fat. However, many people revel in problems with their gallbladder, alongside side gallstones or irritation, that can disrupt digestion and famous health. Fortunately, there are various techniques you can hire to optimize your fitness and guide your gallbladder. In this section, we will discover severa pointers and manner of life changes that permit you to preserve a healthy gallbladder and decorate digestion.

Adopt a Balanced Diet:

Eating a well-balanced food regimen is crucial for keeping greatest gallbladder health. Focus on consuming plenty of entire food, on the side of give up end result, veggies, whole grains, lean proteins, and healthful fats. Incorporate food wealthy in dietary fiber, along with legumes, nuts, seeds, and complete grains, as they promote healthy digestion and help prevent gallstone formation. Limit your intake of saturated and trans fats, processed elements, and sensitive sugars, as they may growth the chance of gallbladder problems.

Stay Hydrated:

Adequate hydration is vital for supporting healthful digestion and stopping gallstones. Drinking masses of water lets in to thin the bile and promote its easy drift via the bile ducts, reducing the risk of gallstone formation. Aim to drink at least 8 glasses of water in line with day and recall incorporating herbal teas and sparkling fruit juices into your normal to live nicely-hydrated.

Maintain a Healthy Weight:

Being overweight or overweight is a chance aspect for gallbladder sickness, as it could result in progressed cholesterol levels and gallstone formation. Engage in normal bodily hobby and try to maintain a wholesome weight to reduce the pressure to your gallbladder. Incorporate each cardiovascular sporting sports and energy schooling into your everyday to sell common fitness and weight manipulate.

Consume Healthy Fats:

While excessive consumption of unhealthy fat can make contributions to gallbladder problems, it's miles vital to include wholesome fat in your diet regime. Opt for assets of unsaturated fats, which includes avocados, olive oil, fatty fish (e.G., salmon, sardines), nuts, and seeds. These wholesome fat manual gallbladder feature and beneficial useful resource within the absorption of fat-soluble vitamins.

Practice Portion Control:

Large, heavy food can crush the gallbladder and restrict its potential to launch bile correctly. Instead, opt for smaller, extra common food inside the direction of the day to preserve a ordinary drift of bile and promote digestion. Be privy to portion sizes and pay interest on your body's starvation and fullness cues.

Include Digestive Enzymes:

If you are experiencing problems digesting fat or have had your gallbladder removed, you can benefit from incorporating digestive enzyme dietary supplements. These enzymes help wreck down fat and help the digestion procedure, easing the strain for your gallbladder.

Manage Stress:

Chronic pressure can negatively effect digestion and contribute to gallbladder troubles. Implement strain-manipulate strategies alongside facet meditation, deep respiratory bodily sports, yoga, or wearing out interests to reduce strain levels. Prioritize self-care and make sure you have got had been given ok rest and rest.

Optimizing health and digestion at the same time as helping your gallbladder is ability through aware manner of life picks and dietary adjustments. By adopting a balanced weight-reduction plan, retaining a healthy weight, staying hydrated, and handling pressure, you can decorate your popular well-being and limit the danger of gallbladder complications. Remember to go to a healthcare expert for custom designed recommendation and steering, mainly in case you are experiencing continual gallbladder issues or digestive signs.

Lifestyle Practices for Optimal Digestive Function

Maintaining a healthy digestive machine is essential for widespread well-being. A properly-functioning intestine promotes nutrient absorption, allows a sturdy immune machine, and enhances not unusual energy. Fortunately, there are numerous way of life practices you can incorporate into your every day normal to optimize digestive characteristic. In this phase, we can find out numerous behavior and practices that let you nurture your intestine fitness and promote perfect digestion.

Eat Mindfully:

Mindful consuming is a powerful exercise that may considerably beautify digestion. Take the time to sit down down down, get pride from your meals, and chunk your food thoroughly. This facilitates wreck down the food into smaller psections, easing the workload on your digestive tool. Avoid distractions together with monitors or multitasking even as eating to stay present and song in to your body's starvation and fullness cues.

Prioritize a Balanced Diet:

A balanced healthy dietweight-reduction plan is crucial to pinnacle-satisfactory digestion. Include pretty some entire, unprocessed meals to your meals. Emphasize give up end result, vegetables, whole grains, lean proteins, and healthful fats. These nutrient-rich factors offer the vital fiber, nutrients, and minerals to assist a healthy gut and sell ordinary bowel actions.

Incorporate Fiber-Rich Foods:

Dietary fiber performs a vital function in retaining a wholesome digestive gadget. It gives bulk to the stool, aids in regular bowel actions, and enables a numerous gut microbiota. Include fiber-wealthy elements which includes culmination, vegetables, legumes, complete grains, and seeds in your every day weight loss plan. Gradually boom your fiber consumption to permit your body to alter and save you any digestive soreness.

Stay Hydrated:

Adequate hydration is vital for proper digestion. Water enables soften the stool, facilitating its passage through the digestive tract. Aim to drink masses of water in some unspecified time in the future of the day and don't forget which includes hydrating additives like cucumbers, watermelon, and celery for your weight-reduction plan. Limit or avoid immoderate consumption of dehydrating materials like caffeine and alcohol.

Manage Stress:

Chronic strain can disrupt digestive function and make a contribution to problems together with bloating, cramping, and bizarre bowel actions. Implement strain-manage strategies along side meditation, deep respiration carrying sports activities, yoga, or engaging in interests that sell rest. Prioritizing self-care and locating wholesome stores for strain can surely impact your intestine health.

Regular Physical Activity:

Engaging in ordinary physical hobby not most effective helps common fitness but additionally promotes pinnacle-rated digestion. Exercise stimulates intestinal contractions, facilitating the motion of meals thru the digestive tract. Find sports you experience, which embody strolling, strolling, cycling, or dancing, and goal for at least half of-hour of slight-depth workout maximum days of the week.

Get Sufficient Sleep:

Adequate sleep is important for keeping a healthy digestive device. Poor sleep patterns can disrupt the gut microbiota and make contributions to digestive issues. Aim for 7-nine hours of exceptional sleep each night time time time. Establish a bedtime habitual, create a restful sleep surroundings, and prioritize normal sleep patterns to assist most alluring digestion.

Limit Trigger Foods:

Certain ingredients can reason digestive ache in some individuals. Pay interest to how your frame reacts to particular food and emerge as privy to any triggers. Common culprits embody spicy food, greasy or fried ingredients, processed meals, and sure meals intolerances. Limit or avoid the ones reason materials to prevent digestive disturbances and promote intestine fitness.

Nurturing your gut fitness through manner of existence practices is essential for gold standard digestive feature. By education conscious ingesting, prioritizing a balanced eating regimen, incorporating fiber-wealthy food, staying hydrated, managing pressure, sporting out everyday bodily hobby, getting enough sleep, and figuring out and proscribing purpose elements, you could beneficial aid a healthful intestine and sell preferred nicely-being. Remember that man or woman goals can also variety, so it is crucial to pay interest on your body and communicate with a healthcare professional for custom designed advice and steerage.

Long-Term Strategies to Maintain a Healthy Gallbladder

A wholesome gallbladder is critical for green digestion and standard well-being. It performs a vital feature in storing and liberating bile, which aids within the breakdown and absorption of nutritional fat. To hold a healthful gallbladder in the end, it's far crucial to undertake top notch strategies and lifestyle alternatives. In this phase, we're capable of discover numerous lengthy-term strategies which will will let you guide your gallbladder and promote most suitable gallbladder characteristic.

Maintain a Healthy Weight:

Excess weight and weight problems can boom the risk of gallbladder issues, together with gallstones. Aim to maintain a healthful weight thru a balanced weight loss plan and normal bodily pastime. Losing weight regularly, if crucial, may be useful for decreasing strain at the gallbladder and selling fine feature.

Adopt a Balanced Diet:

Eating a balanced diet plan is crucial for maintaining gallbladder fitness. Focus on ingesting some of whole food, along side culmination, greens, whole grains, lean proteins, and healthy fat. Avoid or limit the consumption of saturated and trans fat, processed meals, and subtle sugars, as they'll be able to contribute to gallstone formation and other gallbladder problems.

Incorporate Fiber-Rich Foods:

Dietary fiber is beneficial for gallbladder fitness because it promotes wholesome digestion and permits save you gallstone formation. Include fiber-rich food which encompass stop quit end result, veggies, complete grains, legumes, and seeds for your each day weight-reduction plan. Gradually growth your fiber intake to allow your frame to adjust and keep away from digestive pain.

Stay Hydrated:

Adequate hydration is critical for retaining most suitable gallbladder function. Drinking sufficient water permits to thin the bile and assist its smooth float thru the bile ducts, reducing the danger of gallstone formation. Aim to drink hundreds of water at a few level inside the day and keep in mind incorporating natural teas and glowing fruit juices to live nicely-hydrated.

Exercise Regularly:

Regular physical hobby now not only helps preferred health but additionally promotes gallbladder feature. Engage in ordinary exercising, along side each cardiovascular exercises and power training. Exercise permits improve digestion, preserve a healthful weight, and reduce the risk of gallstone formation.

Limit Alcohol Consumption:

Excessive alcohol intake can contribute to gallbladder troubles. Limit your alcohol intake to slight stages or keep away from it altogether to hold a wholesome gallbladder. If you pick out out to drink, accomplish that during moderation, due to this up to as a minimum one drink constant with day for girls and up to two drinks consistent with day for men.

Avoid Rapid Weight Loss:

Avoid crash diets or speedy weight reduction programs, as they will be able to boom the risk of gallstone formation. Instead, opt for slow, sustainable weight loss techniques that promote number one health and useful resource gallbladder function. Losing weight slowly and often is generally more beneficial for lengthy-time period gallbladder fitness.

Manage Stress:

Chronic strain could have a bad impact on gallbladder fitness and digestion. Implement pressure-control techniques which incorporates meditation, deep breathing physical video games, yoga, or engaging in pursuits that promote rest. Prioritize self-care and discover healthful stores for stress to assist your gallbladder health.

Chapter 6: What Is Gallbladder?

A brief, pocket-like frame trouble named the gallbladder is inside the proper nook of your belly. Malice, a experience the liver gives you and permits intently digest food, is held there. If you stumble upon problems alongside aspect your gallbladder, an operation to launch it's far commonly advocated because you require someone.

The gallbladder isn't always an essential part of your body. This suggests that leading without a gallbladder is provable. When your gallbladder is vacated through operation, on the equal time as this will not be saved in it first, it resolves discharge proper now out of your bitterness vents into your assimilative.

Causes of Gallbladder Diseases

Illness or disgorge and gastric: Illness or disgorge and gastric are assimilative troubles that can be carried on with the resource of common gallbladder disorder.

Pain: Pain is normally takes vicinity in your stomach's middle to the higher right additives.

Piss coloration: Dagger's piss can also monitor a stoppage of the same old bitterness vent.

Continued looseness: This is defined as together with having extra additional than five or seven cups of workout each day for at slightest months

Fever or a Cold: This protection is addressed at once as it strength be an infection.

Bitterness: Unusually inside the chair, the Chairs yellower within the shadow can also additionally want to show display a specific bitterness chimney home dog.

Choruses: It can also moreover furthermore display a snag or the usual bitterness vent if the attention and pores and skin have a yellow color

Unhealthful assimilative strategies and liver motive gallbladder issues. If the liver is not beneficial, its aim produces inferior-brilliant bitterness, as said earlier than expressed. Stone can increase from inferior grades and unstable offense. The Stone then punches simultaneously and molds gallstones.

The multiple particular arms that a few thing is your gallbladder are ache. It can be tiny and damaged or instead effective and remaining. In-round champions, overwhelm may comply with to the backrest and thorax internal unique body regions.

Such painful signs and symptoms and signs and symptoms and signs are commonly felt from gallstones, which are not amicably destroyed with the aid of the gallbladder. The gallstones can control the outpour of bitterness from the liver, it definitely is greensickness. Gallstones can also block the pancreas, that could bring about a rash. Hives pancreatitis is an illness with a wildly sudden path. It can want extended period medical institution antidote with multiple troubles and has a tremendously high fatality percent in its most unstable state of affairs.

Usually, troubles with gallstones are linked to the course of the rocks at the same time as the bitterness is surpassed. When the gallbladder contracts to dispose of bitterness, the stones can lie near the bitterness vent. This can be located out as an invasion of bitterness kinks, with pain below the proper ribs. This can release to the right backrest or shoulder. The pain is commonly solid, can live one hour or more extra, after which slowly settle. Sickness and disgorge can show up. Though the pain is not reduced and fever and disgorge take vicinity, we strength be at excessive chance, and medical company can be pursued.

In factor of immoderate situations, the gallbladder is essences. However, the liver persists in forming bile, and the bitterness returns to soak into the heart beat. But there may be a shortage like it might generally be reserved inside the gallbladder. Moreover, bile once more reduces in the gallbladder, so the shortage of body factors may additionally moreover affect the very last outcomes of a higher reduce, liquid bile.

Too slight or too dilute bitterness generates a set of troubles. Individuals without gallbladders typically have issue summarizing rich food due to the absence of malice. For one, affected humans won't be able to digesting crucial gastric, inside six fatty and omega 3 acids. This suggests that obtaining sufficiently obese liquefiable nutrients like K, D, A, and E is hard.

If the body accomplishes no longer supply sufficient bitterness, it can not efficaciously soak those essential implications. Abiding with wholesome accessories preference isn't guide because of the truth, without an outstanding a part of bitterness, the body cannot be inquisitive about this form of country. The most regular symbols of inferior fats danger are dehydrated pores and pores and pores and skin, premature growing vintage, and brittle hair. The nails are slim and additionally crispy and joint pain seems. Basic bloated acids are crucial for an wonderful baronial machine and health, so excessive perspective; excessive pressure, sadness, and reasonably-priced belief may even seem in dire consequences.

Source of No-gallbladder weight loss plan

No-gallbladder weight loss program feeds maintain lived for generations, and you remedy to find out a few No-gallbladder food regimen formulae in Japanese, European, or Chinese cookbooks. No-gallbladder diet cooking is counted toward stews, salads, soups, and grilled meats and veggies. Some models of nicely to be had No-gallbladder food regimen formulae are guacamole, hummus, easy chicken, tapenade, or vegetable salad with soup. Without fiber noodles, any lagging-boiled stir with extra wasted flesh and vegetable, some bean packing containers besides sauce and sugar, a few terms and broth, any salad with out supply-supplied sauce, bacon, pasta or loaf, any tested extra wasted meat or fish, and greens.

Numerous unique formulae can be without issue modified, and the No-gallbladder eating regimen advanced leads, like converting brown rice for and lacking soy and sugar in Japanese strategies or shopping for and promoting rice, thickener soy, gravy, and oil in stir-fries. That accomplished enjoy on any lifestyle prohibits food for an prolonged duration, except diets that ban commercial motion food. We be aware what plant food finished for modern-day civilization, which isn't always an possibility for numerous human beings. Government have to alternate to no-gallbladder food and now not waste food.

Let me say the very last reason why I'm assured that a no-gallbladder diet will all of the time redecorate your energy. When you research the whole lot regarding the assist of the big collection of no-gallbladder and why motion food are so immoral on severa such memories, you're pretty excellent that your choice considers double every 2d you got achieved any procedure meals. I'm high quality you clear up your thoughts; I can accomplish ok, delicious food can assist with my hives and that desire remedy me from the hazard of most cancers.

When you make bigger your functionality, can't flow into round plus overlook about almost all of the fact concerning the No-gallbladder food plan and all of the truths regarding technique meals. And in case you hold kids, which may be sure, your preference is to take into account double in advance than you conform them to the device, coloured food in preference to nutritious, tasty No-gallbladder feed.

The Allowed Foods

Rich Foods in Fiber:

Such as almonds, Row nuts, cashews, and walnuts

Peas

Beans

Lentils

Oats Barley

Potatoes with pores and pores and skin

Poppy seeds

Rice, cereal, and Pasta

Vegetables and Fruits

Nuts, Germinated seeds, and grains

Fruits and Vegetables:

Cabbage

Cauliflower

Broccoli Spinach

Kale

Blackberries

Tomatoes

Avocadoes

Blueberries

Citrus culmination

Meat Food:

Chicken breast

Trout

Turkey

Herring

Salmon

Mutton

Healthy Fats:

Olive oil

Canola oil

Soya bean oil

Avocado oil

Bitter Foods

You embody intended slight food—all of them. The crabs are pretty lousy. Excessive carbohydrates are not most effective horrible for controlling the signs; moreover they exist in what we contact and maintain near at the same time as we in reality need something. The extra carbohydrates we drink, the higher we select out them.

A few remarks are regarding the final amount of stubborn caloric as a way to no longer go out at the same time as challenge our high-quality stop end result. Directly at the back of your consumption, insulin and greasy acids are promoted. You are in the furnished scenario, and no overweight consumption is going on. Your entire depends on glucose within the hours retaining dinner.

As said in advance, the taste diverse substantially once I stopped eating clean feeds. It received me possibly 2-3 weeks to preserve the distinction. My diabetic requests finished almost absolutely. Then I understood to recognize the sour taste of cocoa, wines, dark inexperienced leafy greens, and coffee.

That's why my consuming tea patterns modified from twin ointment and twin candy to crease softy with Stevie leaf Omni at some point of my gallbladder length. Behind, I commenced out my gallbladder food plan, which switched to fashionable dark. My candy fancy changed from chocolate to dim sweet and later to precise gloaming.

Now it tastes bland to my take a look at. Cocoa food intake modified from cacao meals with sugar moreover milk to cacao with best a lifestyles of milky and, in a while, notable cacao. That I idea that is the final object to sweeten only a tiny bit or rent quality a small piece of dairy to take the same lid off the offense. But these days, it brings delight in puree cacao to sizzling moisture.

Chapter 7: Healthy Foods

Consuming wholesome is the legend of a healthy and nutritious body. You should drink nutritious food which will let you with a better gallbladder or other situations—looking healthy food at slightly as speedy as a day choice enables you keep your gallbladder healthy. Have numerous refreshed give up result and greens in your diet plan, and preserve off oily, waste, and method food.

You need to maintain a way of your significance and make certain that you evaluation it orderly. Your priority should exist in useful content cloth material. Before heading to the mattress, you could check your weight within the mild and form in a magazine. You need to in shape your importance every day or on excursion and convey a message of the instructions. Bypass carrying out reputation as this could definitely location a bunch of pressure at the gallbladder.

Keep the Gallbladder Ok:

Hot water pouches are one of the soundest approaches that consist of ever being hired and guided by way of way of using all varieties of physicians and scientific practitioners. They can assist in recovery quite a few gallbladder problems and retaining them. When held in a dramatic internet web site, warm water loads can help in fixing a fixed of gallbladder-corresponding queries. It ought to assist in managing all of the damage from the scenic spot. Again, please shop them in a sterile vicinity. Confirm which you do no longer set your packs wherein they may be disclosed to soil and micro organism.

This is for those probing methods and Bladder-related diet Recipe to assist you in improving gallbladder execution and modern properly-residing. Wish you may admire the Bladder-associated food regimen recipes- permit the miracles to start.

Drink Water

Your body requires a particular amount of water to function perfectly and to preserve favorably. It is sound to assist your body dehydrate in any respect duration. Drink water at nominal 4 phrases in twenty-four hours. Approximately nine to 10 glasses of water are notion to be intoxicated every day. Water can notably beneficial resource you if you revel in keeping your gallbladder healthfully.

Don't Smoke

Smoking accomplishes the gallbladder. Serious individuals who smoke might be conscious of this. If someone enjoys retaining their gallbladder real, avoid smoking in any respect expenses. It is crucial to recognise that nicotine can injure all body organs, together with the gallbladder. It might benefit you in case you said no to smoking and retaining your kidneys healthily.

Decrease Salt Amounts

If eating little salt could not abuse your gallbladder, you have to lessen the amount of salt. You have to limit the quantity of salt you intake if you be afflicted through manner of high blood pressure. However, if you preserve extra excessive blood pressure, the gallbladder could have problem obtaining freed of this extra salt. The gallbladder is liable for ridding your frame of any greater salt, that is greater heightened than the blood deck to your frame. It may also need to gain you in case you even picked the sodium in your weight loss program, which you can accomplish by using studying the Nutriment Tablelands in your meals. It is probably first-rate if you even bypassed carrying different treatment, which continues sodium.

Exercise

It is critical to verify that you are pushing your frame and attractive in some u.S. Of exercising concerning the gallbladder; workout is important and required. When an man or woman is obese and has diabetes, the gallbladder will become sieved. With education, the frame can enjoy some situation of motion, which desire offers gallbladder functioning and health.

The Beginner

The impaired liver method might also generate a lack of gasoline, the rash of the league, inferior assimilation, and the formation of hypersensitive reactions, interior fodder agitation, heightened blood strain, fallacious hormonal corrective care, diabetes, weight troubles, and in fact infertility, in reserve to gallbladder issues.

An unhealthy life-style loads our liver and shows inadequate liver strategies. Loading our liver is, therefore, now not applicable, due to the fact the appeasement liver device is a seemed want for strength and fitness.

If you are specific to the no-gallbladder weight-reduction plan, the subsequent vendors will illustrate why the no-gallbladder weight loss plan meal agencies are so beneficial in dropping weight. And if you are an antique follower of the no-gallbladder weight loss program, you already recognize how cheap manipulate is at denying belly blubber. On that aspect, reflect onconsideration on this department as a reflected image rate reading in advance than mining into the formulae. You will locate lots of in addition troubles based on the overdue meals era.

If you create your feeds the usage of the ones no-gallbladder weight-reduction plan ingredients, you may not attain inquisitive about a unstable guessing opposition. You'll analyze what to consume for every breakfast, lunch, dinner, and snack. You will mechanically eat healthfully. Here's a look at the no-gallbladder weight loss program nutrition and what it will accomplish for you.

In increase, the author and revealer accomplish not signify or certify that the know-how available through this ebook is correct, complete, or gift. The American manipulate has no longer assessed the comments created concerning tendencies and advantages. Please speak for your lawful or accounting enjoy about the advice and pointers produced on this e-book. They are except, as in reality expressed on this ebook, if the writer revealer, any writers, donors, or other sellers, is probably responsible for injuries going on out of or in association with the assist of this e-book.

To create this straightforwardly, gallstones are driven with the aid of way of our obligations. We made nice conditions for them by means of manner of manner of eating wrong food, together with inadequate pressure control, exerting too small, or not sipping enough fluid.

Basics Rules of the No Gallbladder

Milky isn't appropriate for maximum human beings, so I endorse ban it, besides kefir, yogurt, ghee, Fat-free butter, or coconut location, in choice to milky, take a look at goat, or sheep milky. Also, bypass organic and hay-fed on every event feasible.

Dodge maximum nut, and grain petroleum, inner canola, sunflower, corn, grape seed, and soybean oil, which presently account for approximately ten percent of our electricity. Several bloodless crammed nuts and root oils, together with sesame, macadamia, and walnut, can be used as spices or herbs. Avocado oil is suitable for boiling at more heightened warm temperature.

Meat need to stand on a flank plate, with vegetables assuming a vital place. Per feed, servings should be no higher than 4 to six oz. Generally, time desk to consume three or four vegetable flank terms at a moment.

Remain out of flour. Grain may be consumed in case you are not flour-illiberal and handiest on specific sports.

down low-juice fish in that includes sustainably grown or accumulated. Select low-juice fish and espresso-venom seafood which embody sardines, herring, anchovies, and salmon.

Get it relaxing on the give up end result? Their strength is a few phantasm, quality down-sugar, inside berries, at the same time as vegan proponents advocate eating all fruit. Numerous of my unwell appears greater cushty when they hook up with culmination.

Dodge sugar the least bit expenses. That way dodging sugar, starch, and diffused carbohydrates. All strain an growth in insulin consequences. Judge of sugar in all of the systems, as an indulgence, something we eat in discretion. Someone need to think about a enjoyment medication, I advocate.

Chapter 8: Risk Factors Of Gallstones

The gallstone chance elements are meals-related, and others are not as effectively managed. All rebellious chance factors are coloring, years, family facts, and gender.

In-round champions, overwhelm might probable follow to the backrest and thorax within notable frame regions. The a couple of particular arms that something is your gallbladder are pain. It may be tiny and damaged or instead effective and closing.

The Stone then punches simultaneously and molds gallstones. Unhealthful assimilative techniques and liver reason gallbladder issues. If the liver is not useful, its intention produces inferior-first rate bitterness, as stated earlier than expressed. Stone can boom from inferior grades and unstable offense.

Usually, troubles with gallstones are related to the course of the rocks at the same time as the bitterness is surpassed. When the gallbladder contracts to eliminate bitterness, the stones can lie close to the bitterness vent. This may be realized as an invasion of bitterness kinks, with discomfort underneath the proper ribs. This can release to the right backrest or shoulder.

Gallstones also can block the pancreas, that may result in a rash. It can need extended period hospital antidote with more than one troubles and has a enormously immoderate fatality share in its maximum risky condition. The gallstones can manipulate the outpour of bitterness from the liver, that is greensickness.

The ache is usually robust, can live one hour or greater more, and then slowly settle. Sickness and disgorge can seem. Though the pain isn't reduced and fever and disgorge take place, we power be at immoderate risk, and medical issuer is probably pursued.

Such painful symptoms and symptoms are normally felt from gallstones, which aren't amicably destroyed through the gallbladder.

Hives pancreatitis is an illness with a wildly surprising path.

Diagnosis

Your medic will take a look at you physical, which include levying your eyes and skin for predominant shade shifts.

A dangerous way of lifestyles crowds people's lives and directs in impaired liver techniques. Loading a person's liver is unacceptable, as the maximum beneficial liver procedure is to be had for existence and health. The insufficient liver method may additionally generate a scarcity of energy, a rash of the joints, lousy assimilation, and the formation of excessive blood stress, allergic reactions, collectively with hay fever, low hormonal corrective care, weight issues, and diabetes, in reserve to gallbladder issues.

A yellowish touch also can mean jaundice brought on through manner of more bilirubin for your body.

Additional examinations that allow the medical doctor to have a look at your entire frame can be carried out at some point of the checkup. Such as:

Ultrasound: Your coronary heart is contemplated with an ultrasound. It is the favored imaging tool for ensuring gallstone condition.

CT test of the stomach: This imaging test photographs your liver and belly area.

Radio Coverage scans of the gallbladder: This strong scan brings about one hour to complete. Radioactive material is infiltrated into your veins by way of manner of a expert. This chemical penetrates your bloodstream and trips to your

Liver and gallbladder: A test can also display illness or bitterness in chimney jam pushed by way of manner of rocks.

Blood examinations: Blood examinations are completed. Your clinical physician can also define a blood exam to review your bilirubin stories to visit if they'll be

I become concerned approximately you. The problems also can define your liver's fitness and functionality.

Peaceful Liver Life

When gallbladder problems appear, they need to be dealt with collectively with liver problems. The gallbladder is most effective a backpack and a puddle into which liver secretions are rushed. Clearing the gallbladder due to the truth there are gallstones isn't always the prolonged duration answer. Bitterness, which in the long run includes gallstones, is made with the useful resource of the liver, so pulling the gallstones or gallbladder accomplishes not harm the environment that generated the gallstones to arise.

The liver is our number one purification organ, a colander of our body. It additives us with higher than hundred elements and is one of the important organs in our our bodies. The liver is familiar with while we're suffering and taking so cowl drugs whilst we're infuriated, while we consume decaying or incorrect food, whilst we eat too much drink in a few unspecified time within the destiny of breaks, if we hold rested for a prolonged duration, and so forth.

An terrible life-style hundreds our liver and shows insufficient liver techniques. Loading our liver is, consequently, no longer suitable, because the appeasement liver technique is a referred to need for power and health. The impaired liver system may also generate a scarcity of fuel, the rash of the league, inferior assimilation, and the formation of allergic reactions, inside fodder agitation, heightened blood pressure, fallacious hormonal corrective care, diabetes, weight troubles, and in reality infertility, in reserve to gallbladder issues.

To create this straightforwardly, gallstones are pushed via using our obligations. We made nice situations for them with the useful resource of eating incorrect meals, which encompass inadequate strain manipulate, exerting too small, or not sipping enough fluid.

Therefore, assisting the liver is crucial to our method to break or comprise many troubles inner human beings with the gallbladder. We very personal to area in complete diploma to preserve a snug and healthy life simply so our liver cause isn't greasy; that its desire creates brilliant bitterness; that the offense will float voluntarily thru our gastric design; and this is harmful implications can be enacted usually; and any sand or rocks in the liver will soften and be often washed; and liver booths might be capable of restoring and reaching many additives.

Food Power

The predominant robust factor you need to apprehend concerning ingesting ideally and wearing out it's miles commonly assumed substantially better than definitely growing the pleasant food.

All success arrives from keeping a incredible organisation more or less you. Confront it: Choosing thoughtful diet is the legend to achieving any excursion spot. And the identical movements for losing weight. So, in this ebook, you're using to complete your organisation. Contact them to comprehend them well, don't forget them, and then they will bring you for the the relaxation of your dash.

If you're specific to the no-gallbladder diet, the subsequent companies will illustrate why the no-gallbladder food plan meal agencies are so useful in losing weight. And in case you are an antique follower of the no-gallbladder diet, you already understand how reasonable control is at denying belly blubber. On that problem, bear in mind this branch as a reflected photograph price analyzing in advance than mining into the formulae. You will locate plenty of similarly problems primarily based at the overdue food technological understanding.

House, in case you create your feeds employing those no-gallbladder food regimen meals, you may not benefit interested in a volatile guessing competition. You'll have a look at what to eat for each breakfast, lunch, dinner, and snack. You will automatically devour healthfully. Here's a study the no-gallbladder food regimen vitamins and what they'll accomplish for you.

Beneath, we've were given developed a whole chart of food to pursue, and in line with connection, affords a few thing you require to create that feed. What need to you live believing in step with day? It can be superb if you frequently lived, shopping multiple factors and matters that make meaning throughout durations of residing with strong and sensible Nutriment.

Chapter 9: Necessity Of Sufficient Bitterness

If the body accomplishes now not supply enough bitterness, it can't effectively soak those vital implications. Abiding with healthy add-ons desire isn't always help due to the fact, without a great a part of bitterness, the body can't be interested in this type of country.

Such painful symptoms are commonly felt from gallstones, which are not amicably destroyed with the aid of the gallbladder. Unhealthful assimilative methods and liver cause gallbladder issues. If the liver isn't always beneficial, its intention produces inferior-pleasant bitterness, as stated earlier than expressed. Stone can increase from inferior grades and unstable offense. The Stone then punches concurrently and molds gallstones.

This lets in your body to unwind and loosen up and will allow you to warfare off the rash that isn't brought on by way of gallbladder like a nice minor bye product—discharge regular pain of no prolonged intention. Therefore, assisting the liver is vital to our technique to wreck or contain many problems within human beings with the gallbladder.

We private to region in entire diploma to preserve a snug and healthful lifestyles in order that our liver goal isn't greasy; that its choice creates outstanding bitterness; that the offense will drift voluntarily thru our gastric layout; and that is volatile implications will be enacted usually; and any sand or rocks inside the liver will soften and be frequently washed; and liver cubicles is probably able to restoring and achieving many elements.

It will be extremely good in case your characteristic along with your body is in a planet of melancholy and suffering as you check and function via the day, grateful to the scope of changes received to the apparent with the gain of this manner.

The pain is generally strong, can live one hour or greater greater, after which slowly settle.

Sickness and disgorge can display up. Though the ache isn't reduced and fever and disgorge show up, we energy be at severe danger, and medical issuer may be pursued.

Too moderate or too dilute bitterness generates a group of issues. Individuals with out gallbladders commonly have difficulty summarizing wealthy meals because of the absence of malice. For one, affected human beings might not be capable of digesting important gastric, indoors six fatty and omega three acids.

Gallbladder Removes Bitterness

The a couple of unique arms that some thing is your gallbladder are ache. It can be tiny and broken or as an alternative powerful and final. In-round champions, crush could likely practice to the backrest and thorax inside notable frame regions.

Usually, issues with gallstones are linked to the course of the rocks whilst the bitterness is exceeded. When the gallbladder contracts to get rid of bitterness, the stones can lie close to the bitterness vent. This can be located out as an invasion of bitterness kinks, with soreness under the right ribs. This can launch to the proper backrest or shoulder.

Such painful symptoms and signs and signs and symptoms are usually felt from gallstones, which are not amicably destroyed via using the gallbladder. Unhealthful assimilative strategies and liver reason gallbladder issues. If the liver isn't beneficial, its cause produces inferior-tremendous bitterness, as said earlier than expressed. Stone can increase from inferior grades and risky offense. The Stone then punches simultaneously and molds gallstones.

If the frame accomplishes no longer deliver enough bitterness, it cannot thoroughly soak the ones vital implications. Abiding with healthy accessories desire isn't always assist because of the fact, without a remarkable part of bitterness, the frame can't be inquisitive about this form of country.

The most ordinary symbols of inferior fats danger are dehydrated pores and pores and skin, untimely growing old, and brittle hair. The nails are narrow and also crispy and joint ache appears. Basic bloated acids are critical for an superb baronial system and fitness, so immoderate mindset; immoderate strain, disappointment, and cheap perception may also moreover even show up in dire outcomes.

The gallstones can control the outpour of bitterness from the liver, this is greensickness. Gallstones also can block the pancreas, which can spark off a rash. Hives pancreatitis is an contamination with a wildly unexpected route. It can need prolonged duration clinic antidote with multiple problems and has a fairly excessive fatality percentage in its maximum dangerous condition.

The pain is commonly stable, can stay one hour or greater greater, after which slowly settle. Sickness and disgorge can appear. Though the ache is not reduced and fever and disgorge display up, we power be at immoderate chance, and scientific issuer can be pursued.

Too slight or too dilute bitterness generates a set of issues. Individuals with out gallbladders normally have hassle summarizing rich meals because of the absence of malice. For one, affected human beings may not be able to digesting essential gastric, interior six fatty and omega three acids. This suggests that getting sufficiently obese liquefiable vitamins like K, D, A, and E is hard.

In factor of excessive situations, the gallbladder is essences. However, the liver persists in forming bile, and the bitterness returns to soak into the coronary heart beat. But there can be a lack like it might generally be reserved inside the gallbladder. Moreover, bile once more reduces within the gallbladder, so the lack of frame elements might in all likelihood have an impact at the very last results of a higher lessen, liquid bile.

Ways to Stay Well

People count on you currently understand how a producer-based totally eating regimen can useful resource you. They expect that the reader responds to all queries you may have heard concerning this weight-reduction plan technique and that you can begin growing it your self. You finished deliver in case you stand however and are uncertain approximately genuinely showing up meat creations. The number one takeaway is that you make vegetable-primarily based actually ingredients the large aspect of your weight-reduction plan as you carry the primary actions to transition into an definitely vegetable-primarily based manner of lifestyles. You speedy discover that your body and senses pick out out to deal with greater practical, sensible, and top. You can not beautify your fitness; you enhance your food plan.

Fiber

A slew of fitness gives come with consuming lots of dietetics thread. They incorporate:

Standardizing bowel moves and helping bowel fitness, decreasing ldl ldl cholesterol corporations, supporting managing blood sugar levels, encouraging extra healthful intestine bacteria reducing the threat of specific cancers.

Relax and Sleep

In destiny, promising relaxation and sleep will evolve a effective put up to your attempting to find to show a healthful manner of existence. The significance of peace can't be overstated. Among its more than one makes use of have: Need ideas lowering your calorie information, improving your repose metabolism, controlling insulin competition, and Delivering gas for organic motion.

Water

Water possesses 0 power, fats, or cholesterol and is decrease in Alkali. It is the soul's starvation drug and lets in the frame to metabolize fat, helping you in misplacing importance.

Cheerful Mood

A thrilled thoughts-set will permit you to in keeping your vegetable-based eating regimen and identifying your fitness and properly being goals. Visiting as this goals tolerance and obligation, which embody an amazing attitude and method clear up that will help you: Remain stimulated. Concentrate on the ideal areas of your weight loss plan— Confound feelings in the course of your down factors.

Optimistic Attitude

A fantastic mind-set includes you to maintain your food plan and find out your health and soundness capabilities. Seeing as this calls for patience and self-discipline, along with a promising angle and method selection to administer you:

Concentrate at the applicable additives of your sound diet plan.

Confound emotions about your low milestones.

Linger optimistically.

Biological Movement

The fitness benefits of ordinary schooling and physical movement are difficult to control. Playing frequently will tolerate you: display importance, Battle off fitness necessities and conditions, beautify your perspective, Increase your energy stations, and Encourage greater useful rest.

Chapter 10: The Advantages Of Gallbladder Diet

Numerous benefits to this life-style desire, with the number one one dwelling is that you remedy drastically reducing the possibility of a gallbladder assault. Clinging to what's specific as a shared way of lifestyles – so that you can accomplish a shred better studying yourself into particular meals you strength be curious in studying despite the fact that are not confident if they are ordinary – you can start to test a whole spectrum of usefulness alongside your whole body and in conjunction with your method in public. This will consist of gadgets consisting of you will apply your plank– with the insertion of herbs plus the like, within the maximum crucial Haridra, you could prompt to check out glowing feeds and particular kinds across the path from gallbladder-generating particles which encompass summary food. More awesome elasticity– the soundest detail nearly making use of this solution is the tale of elasticity you remedy to finish up with is extensively more all around the senior step might be control maintained within the statistics.

This is critical, as you want to be higher engaged and portable with out the soreness plus the stress of the gallbladder having you around. Deliver your body better food – thru using this technique. You constantly modify the energy of your body's desired approach considerably.

Instead of continuously ingesting the real waste, you gift new protein factors and keys in your body to preserve in shape. Decrease rash – basically like every other number one manner of marketing infection. This is an anti-provocative manner you deliver in so numerous saved meals merchandise and Nutriment you performed acquired.

This allows your frame to unwind and relax and could permit you to battle off the rash that isn't always brought about via manner of gallbladder like a pleasing minor bye product. Discharge ordinary pain – no extended reason. It might be terrific if your function collectively along with your body is in a planet of melancholy and suffering as you take a look at and function via the day, grateful to the scope of changes received to the obvious with the advantage of this way.

You will release the art work and the stress that so numerous sorrows come. The number one problem you may encounter even as you start ingesting this technique is that your choice for Nutriment will range. Like your starting to check objects which have been stuck as "weird" or too antique for your length, you begin to enjoy the type of Nutriment and the form of feeds you may eat as fought to duplication in the food you consume from proper time. Let's convey a desire of what per week of ingesting a no-gallbladder weight loss program approach might be created. You may also marvel if it can be attractive, numerous, and specific, undesirable many fairly restrictive diets.

The comfort of Gallbladder healthy dietweight-reduction plan greater more and better human beings are evolving as aware of the electricity of an right meals gallbladder weight loss plan to help relieve and heal a couple of set up situations which encompass middle contamination, 2 sorts of diabetes, arthritis, cancers, autoimmune illness, inflammatory bowel conditions and numerous higher. Not to mention, a gallbladder diet plan is additionally frugal – specially while you buy close by natural plant life in season. So lets in corresponding out a number of the benefits of on foot gallbladder.

It Reduces Cholesterol

No gallbladder diet reduces ldl cholesterol; flooded starts offevolved offevolved like cacao and coconut. Conducting a no-gallbladder eating regimen resolves that will help you in lowering ldl ldl cholesterol companies, education you to decrease the possibilities of gut infection.

It Reduces Stress

A gallbladder weight loss plan, this is Plant-based totally absolutely definitely elements manipulate to hold a extra multiplied a part of potassium, whose use incorporates: reducing blood pressure and relieving tension and stress. A few potassium-fatty meals personal legumes, nuts, seeds, whole grains, and prevent result. Flesh, at the one of a kind pointer, has very small to no potassium.

It Prevents Incurable Diseases

In businesses in which most human beings display a no-gallbladder weight loss plan style, the speeds of incurable illnesses which incorporates most cancers, weight problems, and diabetes are generally sparse. This weight loss program additionally extended the energies of these already mourning those deadly diseases.

Suitable for Losing Extra-Weight

Swallowing entire no-gallbladder eating regimen food makes it more snug to trim greater weight and preserve a more fit weight with out which includes calorie obstacles. This is due to the fact weight defeat inherently happens whilst you ingest more extra yarn, vitamins, and minerals than proteins.

Blood Sugar Stories

No-gallbladder food plan food manage to embody a set of yarn. This lets in slow-down pride of sugars into the blood drift and keeps you concerning completion for massive stretches. It even offers credit score rating from your blood flow commands, relieving pressure.

Protein is Essential

Instead of constantly eating the actual waste, you gift new protein elements and keys to your body to keep suit. The reduced rash is essentially a few one of a kind primary manner of advertising and marketing and advertising inflammationdasd. This is an anti-provocative manner you deliver in severa saved food products and Nutriment you received.

You will release the work and the pressure that so severa sorrows come. The crucial issue you can discover at the same time as you start consuming this approach is that your desire for Nutriment will range. Like your starting to test items that had been stuck as too antique in your length, you begin to experience the shape of Nutriment and the form of feeds you could consume as fought to duplication in the meals you consume from right time. Let's carry a selection of what consistent with week of ingesting a no-gallbladder weight loss program approach will be created. You could probable wonder if it could be attractive, diverse, and welcoming, undesirable many pretty restrictive diets.

This permits your body to unwind and loosen up and will can help you struggle off the rash that is not brought on with the beneficial aid of gallbladder like a pleasant minor bye product. Discharge ordinary discomfort – no extended aim. It might be splendid in case your function collectively together with your frame is in a planet of despair and struggling as you check and characteristic via the day, thankful to the scope of adjustments obtained to the obvious with the gain of this way.

Gain Good from Biotic Food

People can word it's far at once related to no-gallbladder eating regimen foodstuffs. Aids of biotic embody dandelion leaves, garlic, uncooked oats, beans, leeks, insulin, and onions. You reap appropriate biotic if you consume onions, leeks, or garlic and feature onions on your dish. Investigations have proven apparent impacts on calcium and one of a kind mineral assimilation, resistant layout electricity, removal of excessive blood pressure, colon maximum cancers risk, provocative bowel troubles, and intestinal constipation. Biotic meals even decreases the threat of colon maximum cancers.

Count crucial onions or simple leeks on your boil with onion, salads, plus your life all organizations. Numerous people understand that purple wine is excellent because it consists of antioxidants. But investigations determined out that individuals who consumed liquids of dry pink wine each day had prolonged stories of useful germ of their stomach and decrease lessons of dangerous germ in the middle. The studies figured that when the crimson wine information diminished toxic micro organism inside the stomach, it blanketed a periodic impact at the stomach. It supported the growth of settlements of beneficial belly germ that help your fitness.

Per problem of your whole frame epochs is, from bone tissues of your peel and brainiest, what we eat defines how we decide fumble, no longer cause be healthful or whether, and the way extended we pick out right away. People all recognise the risk of complimentary extremists and the manner antioxidants prevent them. Nutrients, minerals, and Antioxidants that lessen grayness are alpha-lipoid acid, carnation, vitamins D, K, C, E, and A, lute in, crucial fatty acids, and magnesium, numerous B vitamins complexes, terrine, zinc, selenium, phosphorous, iron, and potassium.

Recognize which you remedy not to make 3 generations of in addition help if you supply off the recommended regular expenses of any food plan, antioxidant, or mineral. Performed through fake feeds marked as wealthy in antioxidants and served to bear in mind that relying on dietary nutritional supplements are the severa practical technique. Purchase neighborhood wild and herbal herbal vitamins extraordinary factors. Consume innumerable cease end result, vegetables, nuts, and wholesome animal proteins every day. Turn your antioxidants, and do now not adhere to the perfect give up result, greens, and herbs.

Improving the facts of 1 antioxidant will no longer replace the simplest-of-a-kind one. So, antioxidants need to arrive from consuming patterns and not from a pill. Antioxidants in a tablet are separated synthetic textiles. Still, end result and veggies incorporate photochemical no longer seen in the launch and get in touch with; you can moreover understand them right away. Complete nutrients consists of numerous factors that carry out in adjustment and are far flung greater talents than a complement that gives them.

Affects Ghrelin and Leptin

Weight loss is dealt with with the hormones ghrelin and leptin, whereas cortical plus insulin recreate an crucial element. The ghrelin hormone is the goals hormone, and leptin is the hunger or satiety hormone. The amount of leptin will boom the result, and a reduced organization drops it. Ghrelin stakes circulate up masses before you consume; it way to want, and it's far vital to recognize that ghrelin is removed with the aid of tummy tissue.

Ghrelin then proceeds for approximately three-four hours next dinner. Study suggests that lowering grades of ghrelin influences reduced body lubricant. The ghrelin hormone stimulates the brainiest to boom preference and promotes the economic of petroleum determined inside the stomach province. Ghrelin groups increase because of the reality the body likes to yield to a more elevated area topic. That is why style diets are unsuccessful, and people on a eating regimen their poundage.

The frame wishes all the method food it lived out the dieting length, ghrelin is progressed all of the period, and those skip round to eating technique food and count on that area all the importance. They done resetting their collection pinpoint to a decrease weight and modified to a completely particular significance. They finished to beautify their hormones with a no-gallbladder weight-reduction plan, and inside the lower back of a fashion healthy eating plan, they may be about to courtroom docket.

Leptin is your meal's preferred tamer– the hormone which means that to your body that you have had relevant to devour and lives a essential participant in perfection losing weight. Multiple food can each intercept or growth leptin. Leptin indicators your brainiest is that you preserve good enough power on your fat tissue to enjoy ordinary metabolic capabilities. Plump cubicles do away with leptin, and the brainiest ought to bear in mind that the frame includes sufficient fat, which have to suggest that the body has enough strength reserved.

No-gallbladder Diet and Calories

No-gallbladder healthy eating plan decreases electricity but keeps a belly whole of fibers and proteins that enhance satiety, lessen hunger, and beef up your preference. Swallowing five food an afternoon even includes ghrelin display. Change motives it hard for ladies to yield fats simply the cause of their frame is pre-programmed to get adipose and aspect for babies. In the frame exist no leptin-super meals due to the fact our indoors parcels can't device them. At the equal time, we are able to enhance our sharpness to it. Some meals can assist in improving information, suggesting that our effects can bypass, desires can skip under, and our movements can stay helped.

Processed food disrupts welcoming factors of your brainiest, and then the brainiest accomplishes figuring out leptin signs and symptoms and symptoms and signs and symptoms. The more overweight you are the higher leptin is perspired. It examines the correct mechanical method because of the fact the brainiest should recollect the body consists of better than precise sufficient power stored as grease. And it is an first-rate automatic way, however simplest for terrible folks who devour processed meals. The brainiest identifies its hormonal signs and symptoms and signs and symptoms and symptoms and signs, and the whole lot features nicely. But for heavy people, leptin signs and signs live no longer efficaciously identified, and the brainiest feels the ones leptin moves are mainly clean.

Environmental elements, strain, and lack of relaxation impact leptin competition to a grade. When men and women weight loss program, they eat a speck of tiny, and their plump enclosures save you some obese, lowering the quantity of leptin.

Then the brainiest sees starvation. Anytime you exist in a fashion diet restricts power. That weight-reduction plan reduces and boosts ghrelin and leptin and improves choice. This seems as a hormonal have an effect on that inhibits poundage misplacement. That is why it's miles important to keep the enchantment, healthful meals, and no-gallbladder weight loss plan as a bit of your strength as quick as you hold doing with losing weight.

Consume protein for breakfast. Consume dim inexperienced nutritional yarn-wealthy vegetables. Devour fish. All such food beautify the sharpness of leptin. Practicing additionally complements leptin sensitiveness. Swedish specialists have determined that spinach and some one of a kind inexperienced are expected hunger suppressants that modify vitamins information, avoid weight growth, and sell dropping weight. They moreover sell the liberty of the number one indication for satisfaction.

Meals that lower leptin sensitiveness are you encompass imagined, as extraordinary meals. Sugar is quite terrible. Absurd are not great terrible around controlling the leptin signs and symptoms and signs and symptoms; they'll be even what we acquire keep of whilst we preference some difficulty. The better we ingest, the higher we select them. A few remarks regarding the final part of cussed grease are with a view to run off at the same time as we've were given reached our best end result. Directly while you devour, insulin and greasy acids are promoted. You live in the furnished state of affairs, and no obese prices are taking walks on. Your frame is predicated upon truly on glucose oxidation inside the hours following dinner.

At time passes and nourishing from a feed is used, here's a movement to obese decreasing or use of amassed grease. These capabilities are judged via the usage of blood-advanced and insulin cumbersome acids. No-gallbladder feed programs divided feeds for four-five hours. That facilitates insulin control maximum days. Because insulin shuts down fats discount, dividing feeds will supply that bypass a higher fat-cut price period. Your body chooses not to ignite grease if insulin is to your format. If you believe in dropping weight, do no longer consume carbohydrates three hours earlier than the education and eat carbohydrates inner hours in the back of a motion. That period choice is operated for fat reduce price. The higher insulin you maintain inside the layout in the course of sports activities sports sports, the smaller grease you glow.

The quicker one is the extra carbohydrates be a part of the blood peaks 35 mins inside the again of a feed. Then for the subsequent three hours, insulin slowly levels in the blood.

Glucagon is the herbal hormone harmful to the insulin that starts offevolved offevolved leaking and growing. It's the horrible of insulin, or it's far answerable for lubricant to leak out of the rich booths and residing employed as fuel, and it pulls sugar off the strengths for energy.

Counseled of No-gallbladder Diet

Advised no-gallbladder are every advanced in yarn, inferior in saturated petroleum, consist of lots of antioxidants, proboscis, vitamins, and minerals, are enriched in Omega 3 fats, plus, beyond all, delicious. It's pretty comparable in that way meals and grain are overlooked. The no-gallbladder healthy dietweight-reduction plan we have to yogurt, cheese, oats, and beans.

Beans incorporate loads of protein; the primary difference is thread range, implying that flesh is outlined quite rapid, while beans are referred to little by little, retaining you comfortable longest. And beans stand inferior in sugar, which includes insulin within the bloodstream from spoiling and driving urge for meals. When you update beans with coronary coronary heart for your no-gallbladder diet regime, you gain the reward of decreasing soaked grease.

These reasons are enough for all and sundry to help consuming beans in any u . S .. No-gallbladder cooking is once more remarkably akin to a No-gallbladder lifestyle, although it excludes flour, smoked flesh, complicated cheeses, and pasta portions of the loaf. As all can discover from my weight-reduction plan theories, I moved through numerous steps.

When the palate adjusted because of the no-gallbladder healthy dietweight-reduction plan, I noticed that I organized the waste meal feeds I preferred. Nevertheless, they encompass no terrible things because of the reality beans encompass antioxidants, descending ldl ldl cholesterol plus blood stress, and curd has awesome biotic importance. It is honestly a stunning complement to cucumber-set up salads. The belated dietary techniques propose we trine our existing bean statistics from one to a few mugs consistent with week.

Chapter 11: The Advantages Of Gallbladder Diet Plan

The Advantages of Gallbladder eating regimen extra extra and better people are evolving as privy to the energy of an real meals gallbladder food plan to assist relieve and heal a couple of hooked up conditions which encompass middle contamination, autoimmune illness, two sorts of diabetes, cancers, arthritis, inflammatory bowel situations and severa higher. Not to mention, a gallbladder healthy dietweight-reduction plan is furthermore frugal – particularly on the same time as you purchase close by natural flora in season. So lets in corresponding out a number of the benefits of going for walks gallbladder.

A few potassium-fatty meals private legumes, nuts, seeds, entire grains, and fruits. Flesh, at the first rate pointer, has very small to no potassium. In groups wherein most human beings display a no-gallbladder weight loss plan style, the speeds of incurable illnesses which consist of maximum cancers, weight issues, and diabetes are usually sparse.

No gallbladder weight loss program reduces ldl ldl cholesterol; flooded begins offevolved offevolved like cacao and coconut. Conducting a no-gallbladder weight-reduction plan resolves that will help you in decreasing ldl cholesterol corporations, training you to lower the possibilities of gut infection. A gallbladder weight-reduction plan, it really is Plant-based truly meals manipulate to hold a extra extended a part of potassium, whose use contains: reducing blood pressure and relieving anxiety and pressure.

This is due to the truth weight defeat inherently takes area even as you ingest extra more yarn, nutrients, and minerals than proteins. No-gallbladder weight loss program meals manage to consist of a group of rope. This lets in sluggish-down satisfaction of sugars into the blood go together with the go with the flow and continues you regarding of completion for tremendous stretches. It even gives credit score out of your blood float schooling, relieving stress.

This food plan moreover prolonged the energies of those already mourning these lethal sicknesses. Swallowing complete no-gallbladder weight loss program food makes it more snug to trim extra weight and hold a greater healthy weight without along side calorie boundaries.

Motivation

Nevertheless, one object you must study whilst beginning this diet is a lack of motivation. So notably to select from, regardless of the fact that so notably to update out of your vintage diet, undertaking wherein you need to be in instances of studying and taking element in food can live a extended manner you aren't designed for. To prevent this from taking vicinity and ensure you hold the most suitable choice potential of seeing the motivation you require, we endorse you evaluation the subsequent help for additonal beneficial useful resource in bringing to holds without a-gallbladder weight-reduction plan.

It is a thoughtful e-book, the acute extinction to diabetes is high-quality what you require— packed with all of the records you require spherical seeing the first-rate anti-provocative food. It brings terms and records to utilize it. Still, if you accomplish it, you solve to apply it for pretty a few at the same time as, gratitude for the complicated and comfortable person of the possibilities delivered. Biological Differences Adjusting your healthy dietweight-reduction plan to conflict in competition to this form of scenario is a few element you need to perform on and look out for. Slipping into vintage patterns can help you live in an correctly prepared case. Nevertheless, no longer everybody chooses to control best this for way of life adjustments and extras.

Biological variations that you may force to your strength to begin preventing a no-gallbladder weight loss plan are shown on this record in an reachable-to- understand format that offers you gain a comfortable and easy data of what you have to accomplish, as nicely as developing a honest to address those versions after on down the road. This wise tick list of data from this ebook let you in noticing different strategies to convert your fitness and supply yourself a way in advance in power. That purpose permits your fitness and reliance on yourself as extensively as all people.

This high-quality meals fashion fashion designer and weight loss program helper can preserve you on the precise manner and preserve you from making silly errors. This will describe all the items you require to investigate, plus the most crucial factors of examining your fitness in public. If you want to help acquiring qualification for this form of object, you ought to utilize a vitamins fashion designer; they feature to conventional diets and precise situations of eating regimen life and medical requirements so you can contact the customized issuer you require right right here.

Designer Graph constantly consists of more records and is extra direct to check, and in case you flow into to the manual overhead, you find out it honest to gain motivation. Observe what is delivered right proper right here, plus you want to begin to enjoy the facts furnished at the graph. We endorse reviewing the overhead in case you understand in which to form with this type of item. It makes comprehending the healthy eating plan from a clinical point of view slightly extra less high priced. It gives every different fast connection method side with the resource of thing this e-book to have a have a look at while you require extra guidelines and recommendation.

Chapter 12: Understanding The Gallbladder

It is with super delight that we start our in-intensity investigation of your gallbladder, a stunning organ this is an vital part of your digestive tool and your normal fitness and nicely-being. In this financial ruin, we set out on a route within the route of comprehension with the useful resource of imbuing compassion and heat into the complicated shape, charming competencies, and ordinary troubles related to the gallbladder.

Imagine that your gallbladder is a honest pal who's quietly assisting the digestive strategies that take place on your body via operating very tough behind the curtain.

Hidden beneath your liver, the gallbladder is a diminutive but powerful organ that works inside the historic beyond to beneficial useful resource inside the digestion and absorption of food. This monetary damage serves as an invite to recognize the surprise of the function that your gallbladder performs in nourishing your frame, and I desire that you can take gain of this opportunity.

Together, we delve into the exciting global of anatomy and inspect the specific traits that provide your gallbladder its first-rate reputation. We have a good time its capacity to keep and listen bile, a effective chemical that assists in the digestion of fats and gives taste and amusement in your gastronomic studies. Bile performs an important function inside the digestive approach.

While it's far essential to have an awareness of the internal workings of the gallbladder, it is also essential to be aware about the common problems that would occur alongside the direction it travels. We are privy to the problems that would gift themselves, which includes inflammation and gallstones, and we are right right here to offer compassion and route at the same time as you work via them. Keep in thoughts that you aren't traveling this direction by myself; many others have been for your footwear earlier than and feature emerged from their experiences with easy fortitude and resilience.

As you hold your schooling about your gallbladder, the reason of this financial disaster is to make certain that you're feeling supported and understood. We desire that through providing you with facts and the capacity to empathize with others, we will turn this bankruptcy right right into a supply of solace and motivation for you.

Chapter 13: The Gallbladder Diet Basics Wholesome Guidelines

This financial disaster is dedicated to offering you with the essential standards for supporting the health of your gallbladder, and we would like to apply this possibility to welcome you to the coronary heart of your gallbladder wellbeing adventure. In this chapter, we're going to offer you with the gear you want to nicely nurture and care for this important organ with kindness and attention.

Imagine yourself being wrapped in a warm temperature encompass as we walk you through the fundamental mind that govern a food plan this is satisfactory to the gallbladder. We are aware that making changes to at least one's food regimen could likely enjoy like a sizeable venture; even though, you could relaxation confident that we are capable of be right right here to encourage and resource you at each degree of the method. We are going to paintings together to growth a method for boosting the fitness of your gallbladder via the consumption of scrumptious and conscientious meals selections.

We encourage you to allow pass of any thoughts of problem or deprivation and as a substitute recognition at the abundance of nourishing meals a high-quality manner to feed your gallbladder and promote elegant properly-being. We preference that you may take our recommendation and permit the ones sentiments skip. We place a robust emphasis on the significance of balance and encourage you to take a holistic method to your eating behavior.

This approach acknowledges the simplest-of-a-type necessities of your frame and values the pride of consuming first rate meals.

We look at the efficacy of entire meals and feature a very good time the wealthy shades and flavors that the ones gadgets supply in your plate. We encourage you to recognize the beauty of nature's wealth and make those healthful components a everyday a part of your weight loss plan thru collectively with the whole lot from sparkling greens to remarkable culmination in your meals. You may be honoring the fitness of your gallbladder and embarking on a voyage of gastronomic delight in case you keep in this manner.

In addition to ingesting food in their herbal nation, we furthermore recognition on the want to stay hydrated due to the fact we understand that water is the most important elixir for promoting gallbladder health. Throughout the day, we provide great nudges to encourage you to drink lots of water, and we infuse each sip to revive and refresh your body.

While we are learning the basics of the gallbladder healthy eating plan collectively, it is in addition crucial to understand the importance of aware eating, that may be a dependancy that not simplest nourishes your body but also your soul. We strongly advise which you gather a profound relationship with the food you consume with the aid of manner of the usage of savoring each chunk and appreciating the nourishment that your food supply. Eating mindfully lets in you to hook up with the information that your frame already possesses, allowing you to make choices which may be conscientious and beneficial to the health of your gallbladder.

You can growth a harmonious connection with your body with the resource of nourishing your gallbladder with healthy meals and schooling aware ingesting. This form of dating is constructed on love, care, and compassion.

Let us have a excellent time the nourishing electricity of the basics of the gallbladder weight loss plan collectively, cognizant of the truth that each desire you are making places you one step toward a lifestyles that is not handiest radiant but also suitable for your gallbladder. Embrace the records that is residing inside your very personal body and prepare to start in this delicious and existence-changing new section of your gallbladder recuperation journey.

Healing Ingredients: Embracing the Nourishing Power of Foods for Gallbladder Wellness.

We would like to apply this possibility to welcome you to a monetary damage this is rich in some of healing additives which have been carefully decided on to enhance the health of your gallbladder. In this phase, we welcome you to embark on a tasty journey, in the course of which you'll discover the treasure trove of culinary jewels determined in nature that nourish and keep the fitness of your gallbladder.

Imagine entering a vivacious kitchen, wherein the exquisite sun shades and welcoming fragrances of those recuperation components reawaken your senses. Each issue has a records, a characteristic, and a unique benefit that contributes to the general health of your gallbladder. Let us start our voyage with the crisp, clean embody of apples, a fruit this is respected for its excessive fiber content cloth fabric and capability to beneficial useful resource in the moderate removal of waste, helping the cleansing operations of your gallbladder. Apples are a fruit this is precious for their functionality to help in the mild removal of waste. Feel the vibrancy of your gallbladder as you sink your tooth into the luscious flesh of an apple and don't forget the relationship among this easy fruit and your organ.

As we keep, we stumble upon the unassuming however effective beetroot, a colourful root vegetable that permits the detoxifying strategies of the gallbladder and promotes the proper go together with the go along with the glide of bile. We have a good time its earthy sweetness similarly to its capacity to offer critical nutrients to the gallbladder.

As we delve similarly, we're added to the comforting embody of turmeric, a golden spice this is mainly regarded for the anti inflammatory effects it possesses. Not most effective does this vibrant difficulty offer a burst of taste for your recipes, however it furthermore permits lessen infection inside the gallbladder, which permits the gallbladder's cutting-edge fitness and characteristic.

Our travels have introduced us to the comforting embody of darkish leafy greens at the side of spinach and kale, which may be awesome in chlorophyll and antioxidants. These great greens are a wonderful supply of important nutrients and assist sell the cleaning pathways of your gallbladder, which in flip encourages inner concord and balance.

Ginger, a multipurpose aspect that is well-known for the calming consequences it possesses, can't be forgotten for its reassuring warmth. Its mild warmth is useful to digestion, helping to relieve any ache and preserving healthful interest in the gallbladder.

We offer non-public memories and anecdotes that display the big impact that the ones recuperation factors can also additionally have on a person's nicely-being as a manner to honor the humanity that those factors supply to the restoration manner. We recognize and honor their individuality, embracing the truth that each problem contributes to the overall fitness of your gallbladder in its non-public one-of-a-type way.

As you start to add recovery meals for your food regimen, supply your self permission to revel in the complicated array of tastes and sensations that those food must provide. Infuse your dishes with love and purpose, knowledge that each mouthful not first-rate nourishes your gallbladder but furthermore the relaxation of your being, and understand that that is why each bite is so essential.

We are inviting you to embody the transformational electricity of these nourishing ingredients and to allow them to steer you on a gastronomic adventure whole of flavor, well-being, and gallbladder manual as a way of expressing our thank you for the expertise bestowed on us with the resource of these cuisine.

Learn how the restoration strength of the additives can decorate the health of your gallbladder, and then allow their being involved power to do its artwork. In this haven of nourishment, you may find out the crucial hyperlink that exists amongst food and strength, and you may pleasure in the journey toward maximum gallbladder fitness one issue at a time.

Chapter 14: Nourishing Breakfasts

Welcome to a phase of the e-book this is dedicated to delicious breakfasts at the way to get your time without work to a roaring begin with a medley of flavors which might be kind to your gallbladder. Your gallbladder will experience the delicious dishes that we've got compiled for you, and they'll help you get off to a superb begin for the day.

Imagine the sun beginning to peek over the horizon as you get prepared to enjoy a hearty breakfast in your private home's kitchen as it is bathed in a warmth glow from the developing solar. The air is complete of the perfume of freshly brewed coffee and the promise of taste profiles which might be unadulterated. This bankruptcy is an invite to cherish every morning second, celebrating the importance of breakfast in contributing to the overall fitness of your gallbladder.

Our voyage thru the area of food begins offevolved with a recipe for a delicious and healthy fruit and yogurt parfait. This delectable concoction reawakens your flavor buds even as offering you with critical nutrients to fuel your day. Layered with excellent berries, creamy yogurt, and a sprinkle of crunchy granola, this tremendous dish is sure to delight. As you revel in each mouthful, allow yourself to expect that the vitality of nature's wealth is seeping into your body and presenting you with power.

The reassuring hug of a warmth dish of oatmeal is our next state of affairs don't forget of studies. We offer you with a recipe for a gallbladder-excellent version of creamy and healthy oats, that's finished with a drizzle of honey, a sprinkling of cinnamon, and sliced almonds. As you are taking each attractive chew of this breakfast, permit the mild warmth to lull your body right into a rustic of rest even as simultaneously reawakening your senses.

We provide a scrumptious veggie frittata for the ones of you who need to get your day started out with some difficulty at the savory aspect. This recipe is full of protein and offers a filling breakfast possibility this is also favorable to the gallbladder. Some of the nutrient-wealthy vegetables used in the dish are spinach, bell peppers, and mushrooms. As you deliver in to its flavors and permit yourself to be nourished through them, allow yourself to recognize the concord that each chunk gives for your mouth.

We may want to additionally love that allows you to experience the joy that comes from eating a revitalizing green smoothie. This colourful mixture serves as a nutrient-wealthy powerhouse, retaining the health of your gallbladder at the same time as furthermore delighting your palate. It is made via way of blending leafy greens, give up result, and a hint of coconut water. Every sip will infuse your frame with a experience of renewed energy and freshness, permitting you to welcome the day with a refreshed and invigorated thoughts-set.

Embrace the flavors, textures, and wonderful shades that those breakfast recipes which is probably favorable to the gallbladder must offer as you dig in to cause them to. Allow the sustenance of every meal to stretch past your bodily properly-being, and allow it to kindle a experience of thankfulness and pride indoors you due to this growth.

In give up, we strongly endorse that you offer each dish a strive because it has the capacity to beautify the fitness of your gallbladder further to your every day physical games. Embrace the transformative strength of a nourishing breakfast to set the tone for a day full of vitality and concord. Breakfast is the most essential meal of the day. These meals are pleasant to the gallbladder, so you can get delight from the flavors, take comfort within the vitamins, and energize your mornings.

May every mouthful feature a reminder of the essential dating that exists between the morning meal and the fitness of your gallbladder, and might it furthermore be a celebration of self-care.

Wholesome Lunches and Satisfying Snacks: Fuel Your Body and Support Digestion

Imagine getting into a heat and inviting kitchen wherein the perfume of easy, wholesome food permeates the room and the sound of effervescent pots and pans fills you with keen expectation. This chapter is a celebration of the artwork of creating wholesome meals and snacks, acknowledging the charge of fueling your frame with the goodness it deserves, and recognizing the significance of the artwork of crafting the ones food and snacks.

Our voyage round the arena of meals begins offevolved with a hearty quinoa salad. Imagine a dish this is brimming with quinoa this is slight and ethereal, greens which may be shiny and colourful, and a zesty French dressing. You are loose to test with a vast type of flavors and textures way to the adaptability of this recipe, which can be altered to fit your tastes. Feel the energizing consequences of the vitamins as they provide your frame with gas and deliver your digestive device a supporting hand as you swallow every chunk.

We offer a hearty vegetable soup as a lunch opportunity for oldsters that are looking for some factor comforting to devour. Imagine a steaming bowl of domestic made soup this is full of greens which can be wealthy in nutrients, herbs that have a nice aroma, and grains which may be correct for you. As you flavor every morsel, permit the warm temperature and flavors to permeate your senses. This will provide you with solace and sustenance in your body and soul.

When it comes to delicious bites to devour in among food, we advise which you offer our recipe for domestic made hummus served with crisp clean greens a try.

Feel the satisfaction of making your very very own silky and savory dip with clean components like chickpeas, tahini, garlic, and lemon juice. This will allow you to create some difficulty clearly precise. Enjoy the fine crunch and the kaleidoscope of tastes that the hummus brings in your colourful array of veggies thru the usage of dipping them in it. These wholesome snacks will preserve and assist your frame for the duration of the day, permitting you to experience the nourishment and electricity that they bring approximately for the duration of the day.

In this financial disaster, we will offer you with some beneficial hints and instructions for generating the ones healthy delicacies thru drawing from our very very own research within the kitchen and sharing them with you. Because of the traumatic nature of our lives, we're aware about the significance of consolation and powerful time manage, and as a end result, every dish has been crafted with affordable factors and strategies that make it possible for everybody to put together it.

Allow yourself to revel in the delight and contentment that come from nourishing your body and supporting your digestion as you encompass the ones smooth food and scrumptious snacks. As you achieve this, allow yourself to take satisfaction within the ones advantages. Take amusement inside the manner of creating and savoring those food, data that every mouthful is a step towards achieving your utmost functionality for fitness and well-being.

In end, we honor the transformational effect of nourishing lunches and scrumptious snacks. In addition to imparting you with sustenance, they contribute to the fitness and electricity of your body as an entire. Embrace the tastes, textures, and nourishment that every recipe has to provide and paintings to include them into your each day ordinary in a manner that is every realistic and enjoyable.

Chapter 15: Flavorful Dinners

Imagine walking right right into a kitchen this is complete of the attractive scents of herbs and spices, wherein the gentle sizzle of additives being cooked collectively in a pan tips at an interesting new culinary experience. This bankruptcy is a party of the art work of creating savory and healthful feasts that fill not handiest the body however additionally the spirit.

The voyage starts offevolved with a recipe for baked salmon this is cautiously pro and cooked all of the manner via till it's miles clean. When coupled with an entire lot of roasted veggies, the luscious flavors of the salmon create a concord of flavors as a way to leave you feeling satiated and thrilled. Savor the herbal deliciousness of this meals and the nourishment it gives for your body as you pleasure in each bite. As you gain this, take a second to enjoy the enjoy.

We advocate a sturdy chickpea and vegetable stir-fry for those of you who are searching out a vegetarian opportunity to the meal. Imagine a colorful series of crunchy greens and chickpeas, every of which can be filled with protein and are sautéed to perfection with a fragrant combination of spices. This delicious recipe will no longer great excite your flavor senses, however it'll moreover deliver your frame with the essential minerals and fiber it wants to preserve healthy gallbladder characteristic. Permit each chunk to take you on a adventure through a universe full of flavors and nutrients.

In addition to that, we delve into the reassuring encompass of a healthy bowl of lentil soup. Imagine a bowl of warm lentils, and aromatic herbs, with a hint of sourness from freshly squeezed lemon juice. The lentils are best for you and the bowl is steaming. Not wonderful will this soup warm your frame, however it will additionally deliver a huge quantity of fiber and protein that comes from plants. Allow the soothing flavors to encompass you as you recognize each morsel, and permit them to nourish your frame from the inner out.

In this financial spoil, we percent private anecdotes and beneficial suggestions to manual you through the machine, helping you recognize the significance of putting a balance maximum of the gain of factors and their dietary price. Each dish has been created just so it can be decided by way of certainly all people, permitting you to go on a culinary journey that is useful to the fitness of your gallbladder.

Take delight inside the way of creating and tasting the ones delectable dinners as you begin on this connoisseur journey. Embrace the method of creating new dishes, which incorporates mixing materials, attempting out new flavors, and presenting your frame with the vitamins it desires. Allow every meal to characteristic a reminder of the outstanding flavors and nourishing substances that can be determined in food that is fine to the gallbladder.

As a remaining element of birthday celebration, we honor the transformational power of scrumptious feasts. In addition to presenting you with sustenance, they offer a tremendous contribution in your health in stylish. Enjoy the tastes, textures, and nourishment that each recipe has to offer, steady within the understanding which you are providing your frame with care and selling the health of your gallbladder.

Prepare suppers that are every delectable and nourishing whilst also being beneficial to the fitness of your gallbladder. Allow the tastes of each dish to whisk you away to a global of gastronomic bliss, an area in which satiety and pleasure are not jointly wonderful principles. May every meal be a celebration of your strength of will to accomplishing most green nicely-being and a witness to the pride that results from eating mindfully?

Condiments and Sauces: Enhancing Flavor without Compromising Digestive Well-being.

We find out the arena of condiments and sauces, looking at strategies to decorate the taste of your food without affecting the health of your digestive tract. Imagine that your kitchen is complete of the tempting fragrances of freshly created condiments and sauces and that every jar guarantees to supply intensity and richness to the meals you prepare. This bankruptcy is a party of the touchy balance that exists among taste and digestive fitness. By the prevent of this economic destroy, you may recognize how critical it is to take pride on your food at the equal time as moreover ensuring the health of your gallbladder.

Our studies will begin with a recipe for a lemon and herb French dressing that has a whole lot of zip. Imagine the delightful flavor that might quit end result from combining freshly squeezed lemon juice, aromatic herbs, and exceptional a hint of sugar. This adaptable dressing gives salads and roasted veggies a burst of tanginess, which elevates the flavor at the same time as adding a touch this is moderate and smooth to the dish. Feel the power that this French dressing lends on your dishes, and comprehend which you are enhancing the digestive well-being of your visitors with out sacrificing the first-rate of the meals you serve them.

We endorse a domestic made avocado sauce to anybody searching out a few detail this is each velvety and decadent to supplement their meal. Imagine the silky texture that results from mixing ripe avocados with a piece little bit of garlic, a few lemon juice, and a sprinkling of various herbs. A truthful meal may be transformed into a tasty culinary revel in with the useful aid of including this sauce, which is opulent in every flavor and texture, to grilled steaks or veggies that have been roasted. As you savour each morsel, allow yourself to revel in pampered with out stressful about compromising the health of your digestive gadget.

We moreover delve into the world of selfmade tomato salsa, that's brimming with the vibrancy of juicy tomatoes, onions, jalapenos, and a sprint of lime juice. This bright and tangy sauce is the right complement to grilled meats, roasted veggies, or at the equal time as a dip for healthy corn chips. It can be applied in any of these 3 techniques. Permit the flavors to ebb and float over your tongue, consistent within the understanding that every chunk is raising your gastronomic experience at the identical time as retaining the equilibrium of your digestive system.

We are privy to the choice for variety in addition to the requirement to experience pretty a few flavors on the same time as maintaining the health of the digestive gadget. You'll be capable of revel in the pleasures of taste with out placing a strain in your gallbladder due to the truth every meal is made with sincere, nutritious, and definitely obtainable substances.

As you vicinity out on this flavorful journey, make it a thing to make the method of creating the ones condiments and sauces a conscious and enjoyable one. Experiment with a whole lot of numerous combos, adjust the flavors to suit your choices and take satisfaction in the understanding which you are improving the fine of your food while additionally giving priority to the fitness of your digestive device.

In conclusion, we are able to have a good time the transformational capacity that condiments and sauces personal. Your recipes can also additionally have greater measurement, taste, and strength as a end result, and your gallbladder will thanks for it. Embrace the modern technique and the satisfaction it brings you as you craft your delectable accompaniments.

Do so with the information that each mouthful is an indication of the sensitive stability that exists among flavor and the health of your digestive device. With the help of those selfmade condiments and sauces, you can take your food to the next stage of deliciousness without sacrificing your digestive fitness. Allow them to feature an instance of the tremendous form of flavors and options that can be explored even as thinking of the health of your gallbladder.

Chapter 16: Sweet Treats With Care

This financial ruin will take you on a experience of indulgence as we delve into the area of sugary delicacies which can be type to your gallbladder. Imagine for a 2d which you are in a kitchen that is permeated with the attractive scents of freshly baked food. The air is full of the reassuring, relaxed aroma of candy cuisine. This financial ruin is a celebration of the delight and satisfaction that can be positioned in candies on the same time as preserving in mind the significance of looking after your gallbladder.

Our studies receives off to a scrumptious begin with the presentation of a recipe for apple crisp. Imagine apples, every sweet and sour, baked to perfection and topped with a fall apart fabricated from oats, cinnamon, and exclusive spices. While this delectable dish is baking inside the oven, the aroma will fill your kitchen, developing an surroundings this is warm and alluring. Your yearning for something sweet will be satiated with every morsel of this apple crisp, and also you may not ought to fear about your gallbladder being overworked inside the approach.

We recommend a banana chia pudding with a velvety texture for those of you who've a taste for creamy pride. Imagine the silkiness of ripe bananas combined with the nutrient-dense homes of chia seeds, the creamy goodness of coconut milk, and satisfactory a contact of vanilla. This decadent dessert is harking back to a conventional pudding in that it competencies an attractive flavor combination further to masses of specific textures. When you are taking a bit, enjoy the silky smoothness and the statistics that you are imparting your body with nourishment whilst you take satisfaction in a delicacy this is type to your gallbladder.

A luscious darkish chocolate avocado mousse is likewise tested for its attraction in this bankruptcy. Imagine the silky smoothness of ripe avocados coupled with the richness of dark chocolate, a touch of sweetness, and a hint of sea salt. This is what you should be imagining. This decadent dessert isn't always only a deal with for the tongue, but it also affords the frame with coronary coronary coronary heart-healthful fats and antioxidants. You do now not need to be worried about jeopardizing your digestive health in case you respect each morsel of this decadent mousse as it may not have an impact to your digestive system in any way.

We are aware of the urge for some component sweet to round off a meal, as well as the significance of setting a stability amongst indulging and retaining healthy digestion. Each recipe has been carefully advanced with healthy components, making it viable in case you want to indulge inside the pleasures of dessert on the equal time as also presenting assist to your gallbladder.

Embrace the approach of creating those mouthwatering delicacies as you location out in this sugary adventure. Enjoy the device of stirring, mixing, and baking, regular within the information that you are nourishing your body and fun your cravings flippantly and carefully. Allow each mouthful to characteristic a reminder that you may though revel in the pleasures of dessert at the same time as giving priority to the health of your digestive machine.

In this bankruptcy, we are capable of recognize the transformational functionality of cakes which may be favorable to the gallbladder. They bring a pleasing sweetness to the belief of your meals and assist preserve your digestive tool in correct running order. Embrace the texture of fulfillment and joy that comes from savoring those treats, know-how that each bite is a testament to the sensitive balance that have to exist a few of the sweetness and the fitness of your digestive device.

Indulge your sweet tooth with chocolates which may be nicely to your gallbladder and offer assist for the fitness of your digestive tract all at the same time. You need to permit them to function a reminder that you can although nurture your body with healthful additives at the equal time as indulging within the delights of some component candy.

Sips and Smoothies: Hydrating and Nourishing Beverages for Gallbladder Support

We are approximately to transport on a journey an wonderful manner to be very clean as we discover the world of beverages which can be correct on your gallbladder however additionally hydrate and nourish you. Imagine a kitchen this is overflowing with the exhilarating fragrances of freshly prepared liquids, and that each sip of these liquids restores your frame in addition on your spirit. This chapter is a celebration of the pride and nutrients that can be decided in sips and smoothies on the same time as maintaining in thoughts the significance of maintaining wholesome gallbladder characteristic.

To kick off our research, here's a recipe for mint and cucumber-infused water that is extremely good to revive you. Imagine thinly sliced, easy cucumbers and sprigs of mint being gently submerged in a tumbler of ice-cold water. Feel your senses being reawakened as you are taking a fresh sip of this beverage that has a flavor that is not overpowering but as an alternative sensitive.

This thirst-quenching elixir will no longer best fulfill your thirst, but it'll moreover resource the health of your gallbladder through manner of facilitating cleansing and digestion. We suggest a tropical green smoothie to truly all people seeking out some detail that satisfies their longing for some aspect creamy on the same time as still imparting a great quantity of vitamins. Imagine the vivacious aggregate of amazing vegetables, candy tropical cease stop end result, and a creamy base together with coconut milk or almond milk.

This may result in a scrumptious and nutritious smoothie. The invigorating and nourishing effects of this inexperienced elixir come from its excessive nutrition and mineral content material material in addition to its immoderate fiber content. Feel the revitalization and energy that this smoothie gives for your body as you sip it even as additionally helping the fitness of your gallbladder.

The global of herbal teas, along side ginger and turmeric infusions, is also investigated in this e-book. Imagine a calming cup of hot tea that has been infused with the earthy warm temperature of ginger and the excellent colorings of turmeric. This tea may carry a sense of comfort. This comforting drink now not best permits you lighten up for a 2d, but it moreover has traits that reduce infection and make digestion a great deal less complex. Feel the warmth and the healing powers seeping into your frame as you cup your fingers across the mug and take a sip of the beverage.

Chapter 17: Lifestyle Tips For Gallbladder Wellness

Here, we skip into the arena of holistic practices that make bigger beyond the area of food by myself, investigating manner of lifestyles guidelines and exercising workouts that would assist your gallbladder fitness and increase normal digestion and energy. It is possible to conceive of a existence that is in harmony, wherein nourishing your frame and presenting take care of your gallbladder are genuinely common as ordinary components of 1's ordinary ordinary.

This economic smash is a celebration of the connectivity the various alternatives we make in our manner of lifestyles and the fitness of our digestive structures, data that even incredibly minor modifications have to have a great effect on our state-of-the-art well-being.

To begin, we are in a position to talk approximately the importance of consuming mindfully and the electricity of taking our time to experience every meal. Just for a moment, try to photo yourself savoring the aromas, textures, and vitamins that come from a meal that has been exquisitely cooked whilst you lighten up at a table with your own family. By cultivating a deeper reference to your body through the workout of conscious eating, you no longer handiest make it feasible to your body to digest and soak up the nutrients it requires optimally, but you furthermore mght instill in yourself a experience of gratitude for the food you consume.

Following that, we will speak the importance of maintaining a normal exercise normal and the way this might enhance digestion. Imagine that you are engaged in low-effect sports on the aspect of taking walks, yoga, or tai chi, embracing movement as a manner to stimulate your digestive tool and inspire a healthy float of bile. This is a first rate intellectual picture. Discovering interests that supply you each bodily and emotional well-being may be a supply of first-rate satisfaction for you. Some examples of such sports activities are going for a stroll within the woods or taking part in a yoga beauty.

We furthermore talk the benefits of severa techniques of stress control, which includes meditation, sports sports that embody deep respiration, and mindfulness practices. Close your eyes and attempt to photo yourself in a scenario wherein you may revel in a few peace despite the frantic tempo of your existence. This will help you permit bypass of any constructed-up anxiety and foster a enjoy of serenity. You might also create an surroundings that encourages proper digestion and gallbladder fitness through handling your pressure, on the way to ultimately increase your typical electricity and experience of nicely-being.

In addition, we speak the significance of getting enough sleep and the effect that this has on digestion as well as the body as a whole. Imagine which you are in your warmth and welcoming mattress room, which has a calming environment that encourages you to have a nice and rejuvenating sleep. If you are making getting excellent sleep a state of affairs, you allow your body to heal, revitalize, and efficiently digest the nutrients that come from the meals you consume, which paves the way on your gallbladder to carry out at its great.

We are privy to the issues associated with the appearance of recent sports into your life and the significance of finding a method that is each sensible and ideal on your specific necessities. Your well-known fitness will decorate, and your dating together with your gallbladder becomes greater amicable in case you follow each of these guidelines.

As you put out in this route of adopting holistic practices, you need to be open to the method of incorporating the aforementioned way of life hints into your everyday sports sports. Remember to be compassionate with your self and to renowned that making changes takes time and commitment.

Celebrate the tiny triumphs and find satisfaction within the development you are making, information that each step towards holistic properly-being is a tribute on your willpower to achieving maximum great gallbladder health. Celebrate the minor victories and discover pleasure in the improvement you are making.

In this financial disaster, we will appreciate the transformational ability of life-style behaviors that are useful to the fitness of the gallbladder. They make it possible to create a life that is full of power and concord, with an emphasis on the digestive system's health and the body's commonplace electricity. Appreciate the relationship that exists the diverse way of life options you make and the nation of your fitness as an entire, and accomplish that with the eye that each desire you're making influences the gallbladder's nation of health and energy.

Participate in holistic techniques as a manner to decorate your digestion, your energy, and the fitness of your gallbladder.

You have to allow them to characteristic a reminder that maintaining a healthful way of life consists of more than just ingesting healthily and that searching after your preferred nicely-being is inextricably connected to the manner you gasoline your body. I want for you that each exercising you instill in your self may be a 2d of self-care and a party of the harmony that exists amongst your life-style and the fitness of your gallbladder.

www.ingramcontent.com/pod-product-compliance
Lightning Source LLC
Chambersburg PA
CBHW070555010526
44118CB00012B/1325